The 10 Years Younger Nutrition Bible

EAT YOURSELF YOUNGER

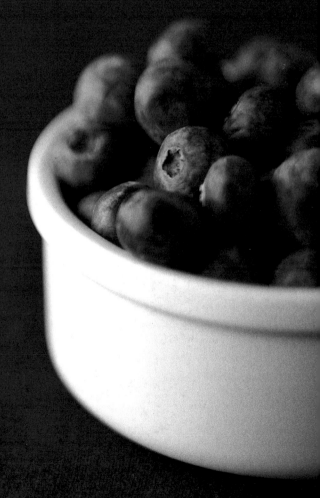

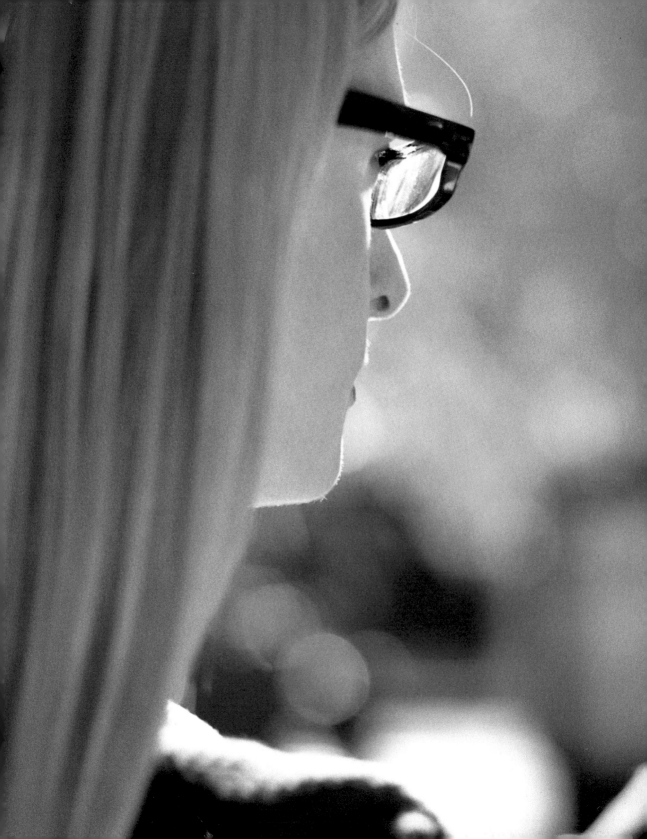

The 10 Years Younger Nutrition Bible

EAT YOURSELF YOUNGER

NICKY HAMBLETON-JONES

Books

To all the friends who have stood by me, supported and believed in me –
I wouldn't be here without you.

TRANSWORLD PUBLISHERS
61–63 Uxbridge Road, London W5 5SA
a division of The Random House Group Ltd

RANDOM HOUSE AUSTRALIA (PTY) LTD
20 Alfred Street, Milsons Point, Sydney,
New South Wales 2061, Australia

RANDOM HOUSE NEW ZEALAND LTD
18 Poland Road, Glenfield, Auckland 10, New Zealand

RANDOM HOUSE SOUTH AFRICA (PTY) LTD
Isle of Houghton, Corner of Boundary and Carse O'Gowrie Roads, Houghton 2198, South Africa

10 Years Younger is produced by Maverick Television Limited for Channel 4

Published 2006 by Channel 4 Books
a division of Transworld Publishers

Text copyright © Nicky Hambleton-Jones, Karen Dolby and Katherine Lapworth 2006

The right of Nicky Hambleton-Jones, Karen Dolby and Katherine Lapworth to be identified as the authors of this
work has been asserted in accordance with sections 77 and 78 of the Copyright, Designs and Patents Act 1988.

A catalogue record for this book is available from the British Library.

ISBN 190502617X / 9781905026173

Typeset in Modern and Meta
Printed in Germany

1 3 5 7 9 10 8 6 4 2

Designed and typeset by Smith & Gilmour, London
Edited by Gillian Haslam
Photography by Mark Read
Recipes by Anita Bean

Papers used by Transworld Publishers are natural, recyclable products made from wood grown in sustainable
forests. The manufacturing processes conform to the environmental regulations of the country of origin.

The information in this book has been compiled by way of general guidance.
It is not a substitute, and should not be relied on as a substitute, for medical, healthcare,
pharmaceutical or other professional advice on specific circumstances and in specific
locations. Please consult your GP before changing, stopping or starting any eating
plan. The author and publishers disclaim, as far as the law allows, any liability arising
directly or indirectly from the use, or misuse, of any information in this book.

Contents

Introduction

As a qualified dietician, I know a thing or two about food – the good, the bad and the ugly. And I know that what you eat can have an incredibly positive (or negative) effect on how you look and feel. This book is about extolling the power of food and how eating differently will not only enable you to live longer, but also look younger. Yep – don't you start rolling your eyes at me – it's true and if you don't believe me, read on.

I don't, and never have, believed in dieting! Just the word diet is liable to put pounds on your hips. Why? Because it's all in your mind. The minute you're on a diet you start craving everything you can't have – am I right? And chances are all the weight you lose and more will creep back in all the wrong places when you're not looking.

Remember what I told you in my first book, *10 Years Younger*? Looking young is about attitude and lifestyle. It's radiant-looking skin, glossy hair, strong teeth and healthy nails. The only way to achieve this is to make fundamental changes to the way you eat – for life. This book is going to help you achieve all that through food. I know what you're probably thinking: here's another book telling me I can look better but only by chewing on 'nutritious' bits of cardboard and eating bowls of dust. Well, you're wrong. Changing the way you eat is not going to be stressful or dull, it will be energizing and liberating.

We all know ageing is a fact of life, but it doesn't have to be a death sentence. How you age is entirely down to the choices you make, in particular the food you choose to eat. Eat rubbish and you'll pile on the weight *and* the years. Yet simply changing your everyday diet to the right kind of food can have a marked impact on your body from boosting your energy levels to reducing the number of lines on your face. It's quite simple really – what you put into your body is what you'll get out of it. Wouldn't you like to feel as fit and healthy in your 50s as you did in your 20s? How about looking as good in your 40s as you did in your 30s? Anything is possible if you're prepared to make some simple changes to the way you eat.

With the food plans in Chapter 7, I've made things easy for you so you can prepare tasty meals fit for a goddess that will knock the years off. Next time you're serving cocktails and canapés, follow my wrinkle-saving suggestions to preserve your looks and have a great party at the same time. If you're battling the New Year blues, follow the food plan to put some vim and vigour back in your life and a youthful glow on your skin. Dinner party for eight? No problem, serve them an amazing meal that does wonders for the taste buds and the anti-ageing effect. Whatever your age or lifestyle, your anti-ageing nutritional plan is covered in this book.

And the secret ingredient to help you achieve this? Well, sorry, there isn't one. No magic, no great secret, no expensive pills or potions – just Super Foods. Like the caped crusader of Gotham City, these foods are full of amazing powers (vitamins, minerals and wrinkle-zapping nutrients by any other name) that really can turn the ageing clock back. I'll tell you which foods to go for (as well as what to avoid) and show you that *how* you eat is just as important as *what* you eat. Make sure your daily meals contain these Super Foods and you'll soon start to see the difference.

Even if you are born with fantastic skin, you have to look after it no matter what age you are. I'll help you understand how your skin is put together and exactly what can make it wrinkly, tired and dull. Knowing how the ageing process works is half the battle in making sure you keep your skin looking fresh, glowing and young.

The writer Maria Edgeworth wrote: 'If we take care of the moments, the years will take care of themselves.' I believe that's also true from a nutritional point of view. 'Eat yourself younger' and you'll not only look good and feel great but you'll enjoy the rest of your amazing life as well.

Nicky Hambleton-Jones

nutrition through the years

Whether you are leading a high-octane, party-animal lifestyle in your 20s, juggling motherhood and a career in your 30s and 40s, or facing the menopause in your 50s, you can still look gorgeous, sexy and years younger than you actually are. One of the most potent weapons to hand to help the fight against that ageing onslaught is what you actually put in your body – the food that you eat.

Our diet has a direct impact on how we look and feel. But what was nutritionally good for you at 18 won't necessarily be right for you at 34. And 20 years on from that, your nutritional needs will have changed again. As we get older, our bodies face different challenges that require a different diet. However, while ageing is inevitable, looking decrepit and wrinkly isn't. The aim is to knock the years off and not add them on.

The roaring 20s

Ah, the joys of adult responsibilities! Getting a job, finding a home, relishing the social scene and enjoying your love life. So much to do, so little time. You may feel on top of the world, at a peak of health, fitness and youthfulness, but what you eat now affects your health, your looks and how well you age.

When you're busy, it's all too easy to eat on the run, grabbing quick convenience foods or even skipping meals altogether. Too much salt, sugar and processed food can cause a range of problems later in life, but more importantly it can cause irreparable damage to your skin. Food needs to be energy boosting, stress busting and immune enhancing in order to preserve those youthful looks.

When you're in your 20s, your skin can look great. The teenage hormones that gave you such grief a few years ago have usually settled down by now, while your skin still has that youthful bloom that older people envy. That's down to the collagen, which makes up 70 per cent of your skin. It's the main structural protein in the skin, and its fibres act as scaffolding to give skin strength and maintain elasticity. Elastin, which is the skin's other main fibrous protein, gives skin its bounce (see page 29 for an in-depth look at your skin structure).

Don't take anything for granted at this time of life. Appearances can be deceiving; your skin may look at the peak of youthful loveliness but, between the ages of 17 and 25, it will start to age. Even the beauty industry starts referring to the skin of 20-somethings as 'mature'.

'If anything is sacred, the human body is sacred.'

WALT WHITMAN, 'I SING THE BODY ELECTRIC'

- Between the ages of 20 and 25 cell renewal drops by up to 28 per cent and your cells divide more slowly so that 'glow' we associate with youth will be replaced more slowly.

- The dermis gradually thins after the age of 25 when we begin to lose collagen at a rate of roughly 1.5 per cent a year.

- Slimness is another feature of youth so be aware that from your 20s onwards your metabolism and muscle mass decline while body fat increases.

- However, oil glands are still producing plenty of oil so skin and hair are being moisturized. Eating the right kind of food will help moisturize from the inside as well to keep wrinkles away.

- The good news is that your hair is thickest when you're 20.

- If you want to keep your face and body looking young, you need to start building in good eating habits now.

- Aim to have a 'healthy' fridge; in other words, something that contains more than a bottle of vodka and a limp lettuce leaf (see page 305 for fridge essentials).

- Vitamin C is essential for the production of collagen and, as it doesn't hang around in the body for very long, it needs to be replenished on a daily basis (see page 107 for a list of vitamin C-rich foods).

- Any skin problems are often a sign of an unhealthy gut. A balanced, nutritious diet is vital if you want healthy skin. Vitamins A, C, E, protein and essential fatty acids are particularly important in the fight against premature skin ageing (see pages 106–113).

- Develop a habit . . . a water habit. Drinking around 2 litres (4½ pints) a day is one of the most effective moisturizers around; it hydrates the skin, leaving it healthy and glowing.

- Avoid drugs, and drink in moderation. Alcohol and drugs affect liver function, immune function, blood sugar control and fat metabolism – and all that dehydrates your skin, giving it a coarse appearance, adding years to your looks.

⋯⇥ *In moderation*, alcohol has health benefits (see page 235). Binge drinking is dangerous and extremely ageing.

⋯⇥ Losing loads of weight quickly may mean you get into those skinny jeans faster, but it can also lead to saggy skin and stretch marks which have a damaging effect on the skin. An 'eating yourself younger' diet can keep the extra pounds *and* the years off; see the Food Plans chapter on page 238 for some fab tips on what to eat.

⋯⇥ Working out and exercising help build and tone muscle so you look sleek, fit and young, but don't forget your bones either. If you want to look youthful and feel good later in life, you'll want strong, healthy bones. Your bones continue to grow until your mid-20s. The best time to work on those bones is now, at a time when your body is still building up the their strength.

⋯⇥ One of the most important nutrients is calcium but many young women don't get the recommended 800mg of calcium a day from their diet.

⋯⇥ Limit fizzy drinks – studies show that they can impair bone development by depleting calcium stores in the body.

⋯⇥ Alcohol consumption can decrease the absorption of calcium so have at least two alcohol-free days a week.

⋯⇥ For more information on calcium and bones, see pages 57, 59 and 158.

SMOKING

I know this book is about what we eat and nutrition, but I feel very strongly about smoking so I'm going to say this anyway. Nothing ages you faster than smoking. If you're a smoker, by the time you are 30 you can look 10 years older. Smoke breaks down collagen and elastin, leaches oxygen and moisture from the skin, dulls the complexion and causes wrinkles, especially those tell-tale lines round the mouth. Smoking creates free radicals (see page 32) in our bodies and deprives us of vitamin C. Vitamin C is a powerful anti-ageing vitamin. If you currently smoke, you need to eat about 66 per cent more vitamin C than a non-smoker. So give it up!

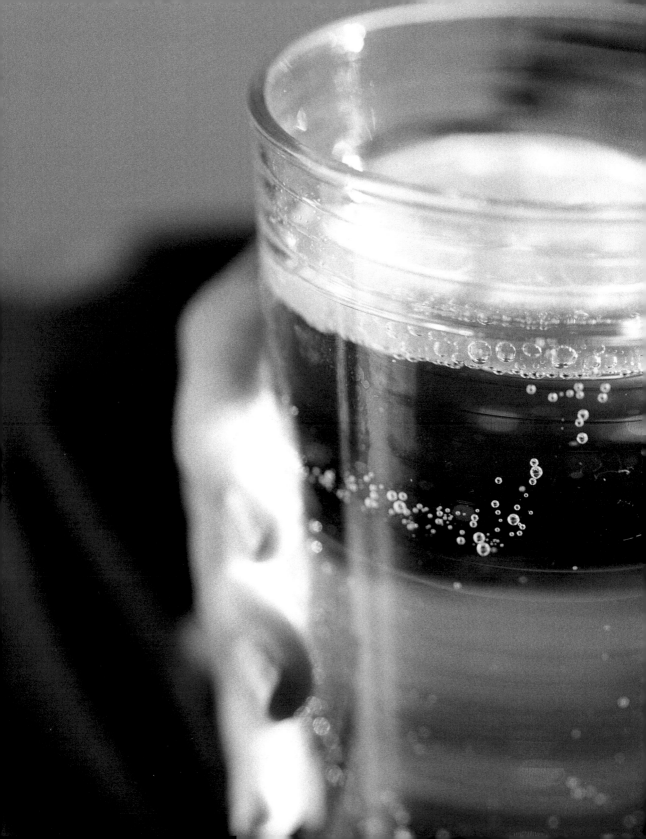

30 something

I do believe that you're never too young to start leading a healthy lifestyle and following an anti-ageing diet. Prevention is always better than cure. Once you've done the damage, there's no food that can bring your skin right back to its former glory. You may have partied hard in your 20s, but this is a good decade to start thinking about minimizing the effects of ageing.

For many women, their 30s are the busiest times of their lives. You are really coming into your own now: careers are taking off, families are started and begin to grow. Everything's a bit more grown-up, with a little more pressure but you still take it all in your stride.

'Thirty-five is a very attractive age. London society is full of women of the very highest birth who have, of their own free choice, remained thirty-five for years.' OSCAR WILDE

- In their 30s, women lose 150–175g (5–6oz) of muscle mass a year and can gain the same (if not more) fat mass instead because their bodies burn energy 2–4 per cent more slowly. Weight-bearing exercise, like brisk walking or yoga, can combat this.

- Keep working on those bones. This is the most important time to stockpile calcium for future bone health – in the 40s and beyond the body's ability to absorb calcium declines and women may suffer 2 per cent bone loss per year.

- Skin starts to become drier as the oil glands become less active.

- Fluid retention can increase caused by fluctuating hormones and blood sugar imbalances brought on by stressful lifestyles and erratic eating habits.

- Cell renewal slows down, so our skin begins to lose that glowing, plump and youthful appearance.

- The battering from damaging pollution and UV rays from the sun begins to make its mark; the collagen fibres in our skin start to break down under the onslaught and more fine lines develop.

- Dieting can still have an ageing effect on our skin; the layer of fat just below the surface of the skin helps plump out the wrinkles to give a youthful appearance. When you lose too much weight, that cushioning (and therefore anti-ageing) layer of fat disappears as well (see page 68).

- The delicate skin round the eyes begins to thin and swollen eyes take longer to go down.

- Be careful how much you drink. As well as increasing your blood sugar level which is bad for skin (see page 50), it can also turn your hair grey. Alcohol drains certain B vitamins, which can preserve youthful hair colour, from the body (see page 93).

The 30s are all about juggling your responsibilities. If you're not careful, work and family pressures can take over, leaving you with very little time for yourself. If you end up stinting on exercise and taking shortcuts with your diet you will only add to soaring levels of stress – which increases the free radicals in your body responsible for speeding up the ageing process.

Teenagers aren't the only ones to get acne. Women in their 30s can suffer from it too. And it's not caused by eating loads of chocolate and fatty foods. It's actually due to an abnormal response to normal levels of testosterone in the blood. Women with a highly stressed lifestyle have higher circulating levels of male hormones – hence the acne. Reducing stress (with exercise and diet) will help bring up oestrogen levels and decrease testosterone.

There are some fabulous food plans at the back of the book which can not only help get you through the year but knock a few years off too. See page 253 for my stress-busting food plan.

So be proactive. Don't let your lifestyle age you. Fight back with a balanced diet, rich in antioxidants such as vitamins A, C, E and beta carotenes to fight the effect of ageing free radicals.

⋯⋗ Eat fruit and vegetables; *at least* five fresh portions a day (which is the recommended minimum) to ensure you get enough anti-ageing vitamins and minerals in your diet – see chapter three for an amazing choice of rejuvenating foods.

⋯⋗ Plan ahead: find fast meals that *don't* come in a packet; baked fresh fish (ideally oily fish like salmon or trout), steamed vegetables and a jacket potato are just as speedy to serve up as a TV dinner.

⋯⋗ Go easy on the salt and fill up on potassium-rich foods such as bananas, grains, potatoes and dried fruit that will help combat cellulite and fluid retention.

⋯⋗ Plenty of water won't add to fluid retention; it will keep you hydrated, healthy and young looking. Drink 2 litres (4½ pints) a day.

⋯⋗ Vitamin A is known as the moisturizing vitamin so make sure your diet is rich in vitamin A foods (such as eggs, carrots, cabbage, pumpkin, sweet potato, apricots, mango, spinach, peppers; see page 106 for more ideas).

GROWING OLD – THE BATTLE OF THE SEXES
It's sad but true. The old adage that men age better than women does have some basis in medical fact.

Because men produce more of the sex hormone androgen, the middle and lower layers of their skin are thicker, making them less prone to wrinkles and other signs of ageing. They also have added protection from the extra oil in their skin generated by testosterone. When testosterone levels begin to fall, which can happen from 35 onwards, men start to show more signs of ageing. Women also tend naturally to have more fat, and the difference just keeps widening with age.

However, there is good news for women as far as hair is concerned. Although women's hair thins to some degree after the menopause (when they lose the female hormone oestrogen and produce more testosterone), early baldness is still very much a male phenomenon, as is the abundant extra growth of hair in the nostrils and ears, to say nothing of those bushy eyebrows.

Feisty 40s

'Surviving is important, but thriving is elegant,' wrote the American author Maya Angelou. I think this is a fantastic description of how to live your life. And what better time to add a bit of elegance than in your 40s? Middle-aged? Forget it – you've hardly started. In 1901, a woman's life expectancy was 49 and a man's was 45; it's now 81 for women and 76 for men in the UK. In the 21st century, 40-something isn't the beginning of the end; it's the start of a fabulous, feisty decade.

'To me, fair friend, you never can be old, for as you were when first your eye I eyed, such seems your beauty still.'

WILLIAM SHAKESPEARE

- At the age of 40, 30 per cent of skin cells are still active.

- In your late 40s, you'll be producing less oestrogen (the hormone that controls collagen and elastin production and moisture retention) so it's important to maintain a high-level antioxidant diet to combat damaging free radicals.

- The metabolism (see page 68) and digestive system slow down around this age.

- Vitamin A and retinoids (chemicals that encourage the production of new skin cells) give skin a smoother appearance. Vitamin C will help boost collagen and elastin levels in your skin, making it look younger (see page 107 for some superb collagen-boosting foods).

- Our skin becomes drier as oil production drops and wrinkles become more defined on our face as our skin thins.

- Skin texture becomes coarser as dead skin cells build up on the surface (see page 36 for some great skin foods).

It's not always easy to avoid stress, especially as most people in their 40s have hectic lifestyles, balancing the needs of family, home and work. But there's no doubt that your body will now cope less well with stress and lack of sleep; see page 253 for some great stress-busting diet ideas.

Muscle wasting also increases as we age. As we grow older our muscles become less sensitive to the proteins we eat which are needed for muscle renewal. However, you can kick-start the release of growth hormone by taking vigorous exercise (a brisk walk will do). If you eat a meal rich in lean protein (such as steak or salmon) up to an hour after exercise, the combination of growth hormone and protein makes muscle maintenance much more likely.

Now is the time to look long and hard at your diet. What you ate a decade ago may no longer suit your body's needs. Hormone- and oestrogen-balancing foods are key if you want to feel healthy and avoid the more damaging effects of ageing.

DID YOU KNOW?
According to the Health & Safety Executive, 6.5 million paid sick days were taken in 2003 because of stress.

⇢ Try a pesco-vegetarian diet – eating mainly fish and vegetables.

⇢ Eat at least five servings of fruit and vegetables a day (smoothies and soups are a great way of eating two or three servings in one go).

⇢ Oily fish, such as sardines, mackerel and salmon, not only help guard against inherited problems such as heart disease, arthritis and osteoporosis, but are fantastic at preserving beautiful skin thanks to the essential fatty acids they contain (see page 49).

⇢ Not all fat is bad fat. You need healthy fat in your diet to keep the wrinkles away and avoid leathery, wrinkly dry skin (see page 44 for some fat facts).

⇢ Legumes (chickpeas, lentils and beans) will help you cope with the impending menopause (see page 197).

⇢ Copper can slow down the degeneration of body tissues which will help keep the skin looking plump and glowing. Copper-rich foods include nuts, soya beans, peas, lentils, whole grains and oysters.

⇢ Drink lots of water; it hydrates and moisturizes the skin and helps the digestion.

⇢ Cut your salt intake; avoid ready-made meals, bags of crisps, etc.

⇢ Take potassium, calcium and magnesium supplements which help to lower blood pressure.

‘Forty-two is the new twenty-two.’

MARTIN RAYMOND, DIRECTOR OF THE FUTURE LABORATORY, LONDON

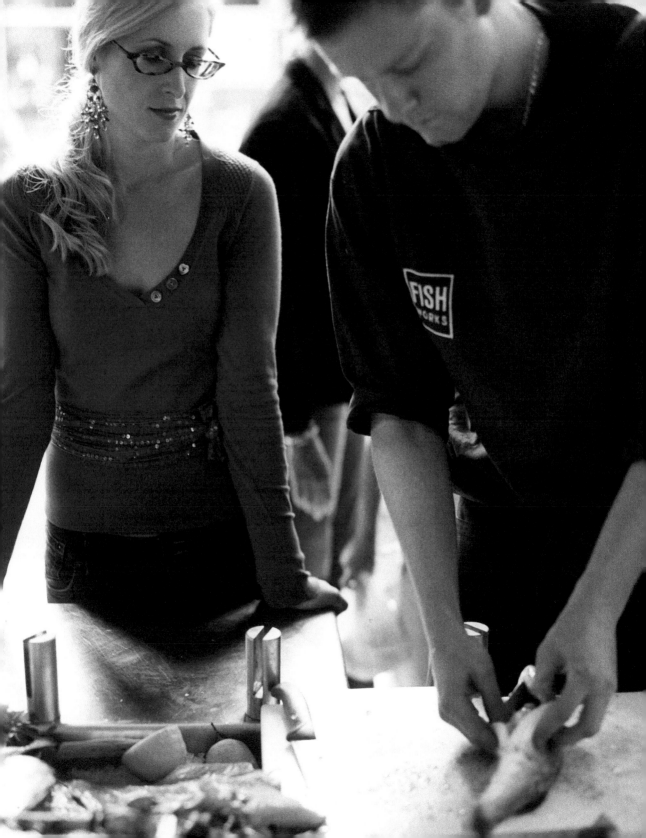

Fabulous 50s

With greater self-knowledge, better skincare, regular exercise and a balanced diet, there's no reason why men and women shouldn't remain healthy and look stunning well past middle age. Sure, your muscle mass reduces, there's a bit more body fat and your body water decreases by about 20 per cent. But there has never been more choice available, and today's typical 50-year-old is far from winding down into retirement or old age. With a bit of exercise and the right diet, you can maintain your stamina, flexibility and strength and still have the complexion of someone years younger than you. With more freedom and, with any luck, less of the lifestyle stresses you faced in your 40s, this is a time to enjoy yourself.

OSTEOPOROSIS
Osteoporosis is a bone-thinning condition that affects one in three females over the age of 50. To prevent low bone density, you need a healthy diet (with adequate calcium and vitamin D), do some weight-bearing exercise, avoid heavy drinking and don't smoke. It will help build a skeleton that will last for life. See page 57 for an in-depth look at how our bones age.

'I refuse to admit that I am more than fifty-two, even if that does make my sons illegitimate.'
NANCY ASTOR

- Sleep disorders are increasingly common as we age.

- Fine lines become wrinkles.

- Skin slackens and is more uneven in tone.

- After the menopause, skin becomes thinner and more fragile.

- Rough patches increase where sun damage has taken place.

- In their 50s and beyond, women's stomach acid production declines so it's harder to absorb nutrients.

As well as being more fragile, your skin will also be more sensitive to pollutants and allergens, but with a little extra care there's no reason why it shouldn't remain healthy and glowing. Good diet and exercise are essential now.

- Drink at least 8 glasses of water a day – I make no apologies for saying it again and again. It's especially important as you get older because your sensitivity to thirst declines so you don't always realize that you're dehydrated.

- Nuts, seeds and oily fish are full of essential fatty acids that help ease joint problems and keep your skin nourished and moisturized (see page 46).

- Eat food full of fibre (whole grains, fruit, oats, beans, vegetables) to help balance hormones.

- For women, the menopause is the biggest event for them in this decade. At the menopause (usually around the age of 50) your ovaries stop producing oestrogen. Falling oestrogen levels cause menopausal symptoms. Women going through the menopause usually find their energy levels drop and they can feel more irritable than normal (see page 197 for the low-down on the menopause and what to eat at this time).

Sizzling 60s & beyond

'Old age' is no longer seen as entering the twilight years, falling into a slow decline while waiting for the end. Today's 60-plus year olds are just as likely to be found on a gap year in South America or enjoying a satisfying love life as their 20-something grandchildren. A recent magazine survey asked 2000 pensioners (with an average age of 69) how old they felt. The majority said they felt 20 years younger and didn't consider themselves really old until they reached their ninth decade.

That's a fantastic reflection on how the more senior citizens amongst us choose to live their lives. OK, as we reach this stage in our life, we lose muscle mass, some flexibility, our digestion isn't quite as robust as it was and our sight and hearing aren't what they were – but that's no barrier to a fulfilling, enjoyable life. And, as Joan Collins, Catherine Deneuve and others like them show, we don't have to *look* old either.

One thing that can decline at this age is appetite. The older you get, the less food you seem to want to eat. So it's important that the foods you do take in have all the right vitamins and minerals to keep you healthy and looking young. Nutritionally, our body's needs at this age are pretty much the same as they were in our 50s. However, activity can decline with age so less energy is needed which means fewer calories are burnt and are stored as fat. The average 70-year-old needs far fewer calories a day than a 25-year-old.

You still need the same balanced diet with rejuvenating fresh fruit and veg, whole grains and pulses, not only to help protect against cancer and heart disease, but to maintain your muscle mass so you keep the wrinkles at bay and take in the right amount of calories. Keep red meat, dairy foods and wheat to a minimum to avoid stressing your digestive system, and make sure you're getting plenty of brain foods – fish, eggs, soya, corn and peanuts (see page 192 for brain food). These are good foods for combating apathy and keeping the memory alert.

DID YOU KNOW?
A woman aged 18 needs around 2200 calories a day; a woman aged 75 needs 1800.

- Omega-3 fats (fish, nuts and seeds – see page 112) keep your brain healthy and are wonderful for your skin.

- Dried fruits, such as prunes and apricots, are good sources of fibre and energy; they also act as a gentle laxative, helping digestion. You should aim to eat about two servings of fruit, three servings of vegetables and four servings of whole grains a day. Don't go over the top, though. You want to be kind to your digestive system – not send it into overdrive!

- The need for B vitamins increases with age. In particular, folic acid, vitamin B6 and vitamin B12 are essential for keeping levels of an amino acid called homocysteine low in the blood. If allowed to rise, homocysteine contributes to heart disease risk and memory loss, according to a study in 1998 in the *European Journal of Paediatrics*.

- Whole grain cereals, beans, peas and shellfish are a good source of zinc which helps to improve memory and concentration.

- We need vitamin D to help our bodies absorb calcium properly. We get most of our vitamin D from the action of sunlight on our skin but because some older people are housebound or go out less often, vitamin D deficiency becomes more common in this age group. Our bodies manufacture vitamin D when our skin is exposed to sunlight, but by our 70s our bodies only produce 40 per cent of what they produced when we were children. The British Nutrition Foundation recommends that all people over the age of 65 should take a vitamin D supplement to counteract any deficiency. You can also get vitamin D in your daily diet through such foods as oily fish, cod liver oil and margarine.

'Many people haven't noticed that old age has been going through a silent revolution.'

MEL BEARDON, AGE CONCERN, ENGLAND

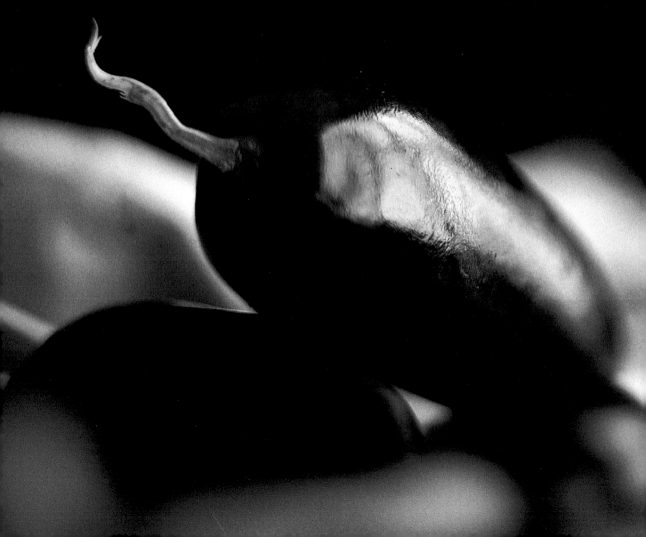

eating is good for you

So many clients come to me having bought a new wardrobe, updated their hairstyle and splashed out on the latest miracle creams, yet they complain that they still don't look or feel ten years younger. Before they opt for ever more drastic solutions, I always suggest they look at their diet first.

Nothing affects your body, skin and hair as fundamentally as the food you eat. Food is your fuel. You wouldn't put the wrong sort of petrol in your car and it should be exactly the same with your body. If you get the fuel right, and by this I mean finding out what suits you personally, you will feel healthier and more energetic and look years younger.

I've always been passionate about good nutrition which is why I trained as a dietician. I know from experience how just a few changes to diet can transform a dull complexion, hold back wrinkles, give hair a glossy shine and boost metabolism.

I'm not a fan of hard and fast rules. Everyone's different and has different needs, but I have found out what works for me and while this won't be the same for everyone, there are some basics which can help set you on the path to a more vibrant, youthful you.

Feed your skin

Crow's feet, frown lines, age spots, the loss of that dewy bloom and crepey, papery skin on neck and hands – the signs of ageing skin are sadly all too familiar. For most people, nothing reflects the passage of time quite as clearly as our skin, and nothing gives away our age quite as obviously as our face. When meeting someone new, everyone automatically focuses on their face and it usually provides a very accurate barometer of how well we are looking after ourselves, how good our diet is and just how healthy we really are.

Ageing skin – what happens

⋯⟩ With ageing, the outer skin layer, or epidermis, thins even though the actual number of cell layers remains the same.

⋯⟩ The number of pigment-producing cells, or melanocytes, which are found in the lower part of the epidermis decreases but those remaining clump together and increase in size. As a result, skin looks thinner and paler, and sunspots appear in sun-damaged areas.

⋯⟩ The dermis, or inner layer of skin, mainly consists of connective tissue, in particular collagen and elastin. When clinicians talk about living skin, they are referring to the dermis.

⋯⟩ The dermis basically supports the epidermis, supplying it with everything it needs to provide an effective barrier. It is also vital for the skin's immune and repair systems.

⋯⟩ Roughly 95 per cent of the dermis is made up of collagen and 3 per cent of elastin.

⋯⟩ Hair follicles, sebaceous (oil) and sweat glands are also present in this layer.

⋯⟩ As we age, the loss of collagen and elastin from the dermis reduces the skin's strength and elasticity. This process is called elastosis and is particularly obvious in sun-exposed areas where skin can take on a dry, weathered, leathery appearance.

⋯⟩ Skin produces less oil as it ages, leaving it dry and more prone to wrinkles.

⋯⟩ The subcutaneous fat layer below the dermis also thins, reducing its ability to maintain temperature and cushion the skin against injury. This is particularly noticeable in anyone who is underweight.

Scientists are increasingly clear about what causes skin to age and the main culprits are:

1 Free radical damage which also depletes collagen and elastin, and slows the rate of cell renewal.
2 Cell degeneration through natural deterioration.
3 Skin inflammation and irritation from pollution, sunlight and other allergens which gradually wear away the skin's immune system.
4 Hormone changes.

Added to these factors is the hand your genes has dealt you. It used to be said that to see how well a woman will age, you should look at her mother. This is true to a point, but experts are being challenged to find ways to tackle these inherited genes and discover how to prevent or delay them from switching on the signs of ageing before they become apparent in our skin.

'Approximately 25 per cent of how a person ages is inherited from parents. Stress, environment, nutrition, lifestyle and immunity play an additional role.'

PROFESSOR THOMAS KIRKWOOD, UNIVERSITY OF NEWCASTLE AND DIRECTOR OF THE INSTITUTE OF AGEING AND HEALTH

There is growing agreement that the best way forward is to combat skin ageing from the inside as well as the outside, which basically means a combination of topical skincare and nutrition.

I'm going to assume you've read my first book *10 Years Younger* and so already know how vital it is to:

···> Follow a good, daily skincare routine, which takes account of your changing needs as you age.

···> Always protect your skin against sun damage, which means using products with a built-in SPF all year round with specific high-factor protection in the summer.

···> Stop smoking – nothing ages skin faster and a combination of smoke and sun worship is a disaster if you don't want your skin to look years older than your true age.

But ... however much care you take of your skin, however much you spend on the latest high-tech skincare products, it will be pointless if you don't also take care of your diet and really think about the foods you eat and the effects they may be having on your body.

DID YOU KNOW?

Many of the ingredients listed in anti-ageing creams are exactly the same things you should be eating – in particular look out for vitamins A, C and E, minerals such as selenium, essential oils and supplements like co-enzyme Q10 and green tea extract.

Combating the signs of ageing

Free radical damage

The problem:

---》 To see free radical damage, or oxidation, in action you only have to watch what happens to a cut slice of apple – it quickly turns brown as the exposed cells react with oxygen in the atmosphere. Exactly the same process takes place in your body and skin (albeit with slightly different results). Sunlight, smoking, pollution, toxins in the air we breathe and food we eat all work to accelerate the damage and trigger more free radicals.

---》 Free radicals also deplete collagen and elastin, making the fibres tougher and causing them to shrink. It is collagen, supported by hyaluronic acid (see page 37), which gives youthful skin its plumpness and a lack of it leaves skin looking dry and as if it has lost its spring. Ultimately the loss of collagen leads to sagging skin and turns fine lines into wrinkles and folds.

---》 Free radicals affect the skin's pigmentation, causing sunspots and the hyperpigmentation that is associated with age and over-exposure to sunlight. Over time, free radicals slow the body's ability to generate new skin cells and skin appears noticeably older as new, plump, firm cells don't replace the old, shrivelled ones.

The anti-ageing solution:

---》 Don't despair, it's not all bad news. We can defend ourselves. Antioxidants work to minimize the damage caused by free radicals and to keep cells healthy. They are already present in our bodies and also in some foods, and so one obvious solution is to boost our intake by eating a diet rich in antioxidants.

DID YOU KNOW?
Free radicals are so called because they are missing a vital molecule which leads them to attack and in turn damage other cells in a bid to reacquire their missing molecule.

DID YOU KNOW?
Miriam Stoppard calculates that the face of a 20-a-day smoker ages 14 years for every 10 years of smoking. Another sobering fact is that smokers in their 40s often have as many wrinkles as non-smokers in their 60s. 》 Some scientists believe that sunlight accounts for up to 80 per cent of the symptoms of ageing in the skin.

Antioxidants

Antioxidants include vitamins, minerals and other compounds in food. The biggest group of antioxidants are flavonoids – these are basically the phytochemicals which give fruits and vegetables their colour and taste. The purple-blue-red-orange spectrum contains the most antioxidant-rich fruits and vegetables.

Antioxidant-rich fruits include:

- Blackberries
- Blueberries
- Cranberries
- Grapes
- Peaches
- Plums

Antioxidant-rich vegetables include:

- Artichokes
- Asparagus
- Aubergines
- Beans
- Broccoli
- Potatoes
- Spinach
- Sweet potatoes

Antioxidant-rich nuts include:

- Hazelnuts
- Pecans
- Walnuts

However, even though a food may be very high in antioxidants, a more important factor is what happens when it is eaten as some compounds are not easily digested and absorbed. Many need another enzyme present to help the body absorb it. The best advice is to eat a variety of foods. Each is unique, some with more vitamins or fibre than others, and by eating a mixture you make sure you can enhance what you're taking in nutritionally.

DID YOU KNOW?
Don't assume raw is always best. Sometimes cooking improves the absorption of flavonoids, for instance lycopene in tomatoes.

DID YOU KNOW?
An antioxidant called resveratrol which is found in red grapes, red grape juice and red wine seems to affect ageing, allowing cells to live longer. It is also thought to offset the dangers of cancer, heart disease and Alzheimer's. » Hollywood celebrities are drinking pomegranate juice – it is a good source of ellagic acid which boosts the skin's natural defences against sun damage. » Just one cupful of berries a day provides you with all the antioxidants you need. Alternately, just seven prunes will do the same.

Antioxidant vitamins

As well as being powerful antioxidants counteracting the ageing effects of free radicals, these vitamins all have specific effects that can help your skin look younger.

Vitamin A

⇢ Essential for skin maintenance and repair.
⇢ Dermal cells in the epidermis, or outer layer of skin, lose moisture as they move towards the surface. They become harder and flatter as levels of a protein called keratin become more concentrated. Vitamin A helps to control this concentration.
⇢ A lack of vitamin A will result in a dry, flaky, rough complexion and pimples.
⇢ Recommended daily allowance (RDA) is 800mcg.
⇢ Over-consumption of supplements can be toxic. However, when eaten naturally as beta carotene in food, it is not toxic as the body regulates how much is converted to vitamin A.

Best food sources:
Liver, dairy foods, eggs, oily fish and brightly-coloured fruits and vegetables where it's present as beta carotene, especially leafy greens and broccoli, carrots, sweet potatoes, apricots, cantaloupe melon, pumpkin and squash.

Vitamin C

⇢ Powerful antiviral and antibacterial action.
⇢ Boosts collagen production by converting the amino acid proline into hydroxyproline. Without vitamin C, skin would have no collagen.
⇢ Boosts skin renewal and regrowth.
⇢ Helps the body absorb vitamins and minerals.
⇢ RDA is 1–2g.

Best food sources:
Citrus fruits, kiwi fruit, strawberries, guava, blackcurrants, sweet potatoes, peppers, leafy green veg, tomatoes.

Vitamin E

⇢ Stimulates cell growth, skin healing and reduces inflammation.
⇢ Works well with vitamin C, making it even more effective against free radicals.
⇢ One study suggested that a combination of vitamins C and E might reduce skin reactions to sunburn (although any protection would be far less than from a sunscreen).
⇢ RDA is 10mg.

Best food sources:
Wheatgerm and oil, nuts, sunflower seeds, vegetable oils, olives, avocados, blackberries, fish, shellfish, tomatoes, sweet potatoes, leafy green veg, whole grains.

Antioxidant minerals

Selenium

⟶ Essential for the production of glutathione, the body's free-radical scavenger.
⟶ Works best when eaten with other foods containing vitamins A, C and E.
⟶ There is no official RDA but nutrition experts agree we need a minimum of 70mg. In Britain, most people only average around 30mg.

Best food sources:
Brazil nuts, seaweed, lean meat, fish (including shellfish), cashews, walnuts, sunflower seeds, whole wheat bread and cereals, cheese, eggs.

Zinc

⟶ Essential for the production of new, healthy epidermal growth.
⟶ A lack of zinc causes poor skin healing and stretch marks.
⟶ A deficiency is also associated with a wide variety of skin complaints, including acne and eczema.
⟶ RDA is 15mg.

Best food sources:
Pecan nuts, pumpkin seeds, sardines, brown rice, cheese, lentils, rye.

⟶ **Silica** is another useful antioxidant – see page 42.
⟶ **Essential fatty acids and Omega-3 oils** are also very powerful antioxidants. For more information, see page 46.

DID YOU KNOW?
Eating just four or five brazil nuts a day will give you all the selenium your body needs.

Wrinkle-zapping foods

The Human Nutrition Research Centre in Boston conducted studies to measure levels of antioxidants in food. The test is known as Oxygen Radical Absorbence Capacity, or ORAC. Results were put together to compile a list of the top-scoring wrinkle-zapping fruit and vegetables. It is thought that it is the combination of vitamins, minerals and flavonoids which makes these foods so effective – not just at combating skin ageing but also in protecting against arthritis, improving circulation, memory and brain function and in reducing the risk of some cancers and heart disease.

Top-scoring ORAC foods

Fruit	**Vegetables**
⋯▸ Blackberries	⋯▸ Alfalfa sprouts
⋯▸ Blueberries	⋯▸ Aubergines
⋯▸ Cherries	⋯▸ Beetroot
⋯▸ Kiwi fruit	⋯▸ Broccoli
⋯▸ Oranges	⋯▸ Brussels sprouts
⋯▸ Pink grapefruit	⋯▸ Corn
⋯▸ Plums	⋯▸ Kale
⋯▸ Prunes	⋯▸ Onions
⋯▸ Raisins	⋯▸ Red peppers
⋯▸ Raspberries	⋯▸ Spinach
⋯▸ Red grapes	
⋯▸ Strawberries	

DID YOU KNOW?
Although strawberries scored higher in the ORAC test, eating spinach resulted in a greater rise in blood antioxidant levels.

DID YOU KNOW?
Recent years have seen a huge growth in the number of products labelled as antioxidant-rich and specifically marketed as anti-ageing. 'Antioxidant vitamins have long been added to food products but companies are making a bigger deal of this now,' says Lucy Cornford, a research analyst at Mintel. 'Companies are really working on the assumption that the consumer knows about antioxidants and links them to anti-ageing.'

Hyaluronic acid – skin's super-moisturizer

···> Hyaluronic acid occurs naturally in the skin and helps retain natural moisture.

···> It is the skin's most effective moisturizing agent. Each molecule holds 214 molecules of water.

···> Not only does it retain water, it also supplies nutrients and removes waste.

···> Sadly, over time, the natural process of ageing and environmental factors like sunlight and pollution deplete the amounts present in the skin. In other words, just when we need it most, there is less available.

···> Hyaluronic acid is the cement of connective tissue. It supports collagen and elastin in the dermis.

···> Hyaluronic acid effectively moisturizes the skin from the inside.

···> Researchers claim it can smooth wrinkles and have called it an 'internal cosmetic'.

The levels of hyaluronic acid present in the body can be affected by many factors:

···> Genetic makeup may play a part.

···> Zinc and magnesium deficiencies are associated with hyaluronic acid abnormalities.

···> Clinical tests also suggest a link between zinc deficiency and low levels of both hyaluronic acid and collagen.

···> Protein deficiency may also lead to low levels of the acid in skin.

···> Oestrogen boosts activity.

···> Smoking degrades hyaluronic acid.

Best food sources:
Beans, pulses, starchy root vegetables, chicken broth where bones and skin have been used as the basis of the soup.

DID YOU KNOW?
Dr Toyosuke Kemori, a doctor in the Japanese village of Yuzuri Hara, 2 hours from Tokyo, believes regional starchy vegetables, in particular a type of sweet potato and a potato root called imoji, stimulate the production of hyaluronic acid and are responsible for the villagers' longevity and youthful skin. 'I have never seen anyone suffer from skin cancer here,' he comments, adding, 'I have seen a woman in her 90s with spotless skin.'

DID YOU KNOW?
Hyaluronic acid can be used as a topical skin treatment. Synthetic hyaluronic acid is used to treat lines and scars and improve facial contours. It's a safe alternative to collagen.

Cell degeneration

The problem:

An average adult has around 300 million skin cells. There is an outer layer called the epidermis which is constantly growing from the bottom layer up, a middle fibrous layer called the dermis, and beneath this a layer of subcutaneous fat. Like all cells, those in the skin are constantly renewing themselves but with each reproduction cycle, the cells go through some alteration or deterioration and, as the cells deteriorate, we age.

DNA and RNA are the basic building blocks of life. All the information our bodies need to grow and function is stored in DNA in the cell nucleus. This information code is then passed on to RNA and finally to the various enzymes and proteins which actually make the body work. Both DNA and RNA are made from nucleic acid bases which are usually made from the amino acids, vitamin co-factors and enzymes in our diet. But recent studies have shown that the body is not always able to produce enough DNA and RNA to regenerate and repair cells properly. Stress in particular affects the body's ability to replace cells quickly.

Fact file

⋯⇥ Nucleic acids rejuvenate and feed deteriorating cells.

⋯⇥ DNA and RNA are our body's nucleic acids.

⋯⇥ If DNA stops functioning properly and does not pass on messages to RNA, new cell generation in the body simply stops.

The anti-ageing solution:

Research in the US suggests that by keeping the body well fed with nucleic acids, you can look and feel between eight and 12 years younger than your actual age. You will not only have more energy but your skin will look and feel healthier and more youthful.

Although the body produces its own nucleic acids they are broken down very quickly and need to be supplemented nutritionally if we want to slow the ageing process.

Nucleic acid-rich food

⋯⇥ The body needs between 1–1.5g a day.

⋯⇥ **Best food sources:**
Asparagus, spinach, mushrooms, onions, wheatgerm, bran, oatmeal, some forms of yeast, fish (in particular oily fish like salmon and sardines), chicken liver.

DID YOU KNOW?
It normally takes between 52 and 75 days for a complete renewal cycle from the development of new skin cells until they are shed.

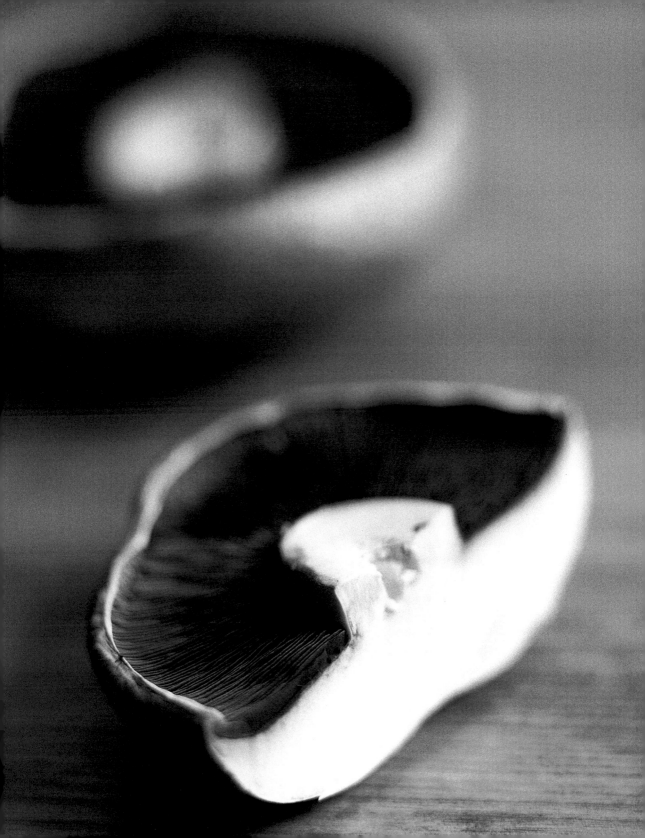

Skin inflammation and irritation

The problem:

Attacks on the immune system, pollution, sunlight, the food we eat and harsh skin care products all combine to assault and stress skin causing inflammation and irritation. Everyday factors such as stress and lack of sleep make the problem worse.

Dr Nicholas Perricone, skincare guru and author of *The Wrinkle Cure* and *The Perricone Prescription*, believes the connection between inflammation and ageing is fundamental. He states, 'When I looked at a biopsy of skin that showed clinical signs of ageing, inflammation was present. Yet skin that showed no clinical signs of ageing showed no inflammation.'

The anti-ageing solution:

Free radical damage is an important factor causing skin inflammation and so again, boosting your intake of antioxidant-rich foods is vital. But there are other equally important adjustments you can make nutritionally which will help prevent wrinkles.

Immune boosters

When skin is stressed it looks red and inflamed, whether the cause is sunburn or a reaction to food or a skin cream, and there's no doubt that stressed skin ages faster. For skin to repair the damage the immune system must function efficiently. A healthy immune system is a good step towards general fitness with your body as a whole performing at the peak of its capacity.

If your immune system is weak, it will affect your skin's ability to act as a barrier to pollution and other external factors, leaving it prone to inflammation and irritation. In addition, the fact that your body is not performing as effectively as it should, with the liver, kidneys and bowels all excreting waste efficiently, means your skin will have to work extra hard to expel excess toxins.

(For more information on immune-boosting foods, see pages 247.)

Vital vitamins

B-complex vitamins

⇢ These include vitamins B6 pyridoxine, B12 cyanocobalamin, B1 thiamin, B2 riboflavin, B3 niacin and folic acid.
⇢ Most are co-enzymes which means they work together with other compounds to make sure vital body processes take place.
⇢ They are particularly important for healthy skin, nerves and brain and essential for many chemical reactions, allowing the body to use proteins and amino acids.
⇢ B vitamins help balance hormones.
⇢ They play an important role in white blood cell activity and the production of antibodies. This means they are vital for immune function and fighting infection.
⇢ RDA varies for each B vitamin: B1 1.5mg, B2 1.7mg, B3 20mg, B6 2mg, B12 6mcg, Folic Acid 400mcg.
⇢ In skincare, vitamin B is effective in treating acne and relieving dry, itchy skin.
⇢ Too much sugar, processed food, alcohol, stress, pollution and illness can all lead to a deficiency of B vitamins.

Best food sources:
Spinach, broccoli, asparagus, tomato juice, legumes, melons, oranges, lentils, beans, peanuts, almonds, hazelnuts, wheatgerm, whole grains, eggs, fish, shellfish, liver, chicken, natural yogurt, soya.

Vitamin D

⇢ We need more vitamin D as we age.
⇢ It plays an important role in skin cell metabolism and growth.
⇢ Vitamin D is essential for the proper absorption of calcium in the body.
⇢ This vitamin may be useful in treating the itching and flakiness associated with psoriasis.
⇢ RDA is 400iu.

Best sources:
Most of our vitamin D is produced through exposure to sunlight; however, over the age of 65 we tend not to get enough vitamin D from the sun (this doesn't, of course, mean that you should lie in the sun without sun protection). Food sources include oily fish and fish oils, milk, egg yolks, liver.

Mighty minerals

Silica

This is one of the most abundant minerals on earth – it is found in sand, flint, natural water supplies and in the earth's crust. It is also present in our bodies in skin, hair and nails. Many people are not aware of its existence, yet it has powerful anti-ageing properties.

The facts:
- Silica is essential for the formation of white blood cells.
- It improves immune function.
- It also soothes, protects, reduces inflammation, removes toxins and starts the healing process.
- Silica is important for the utilization of several other vitamins and minerals.
- Silica regenerates skin, working with vitamin C and prompting the production of collagen and elastin.
- Clinical trials have shown that silica actually helps to thicken and boost the dermis, improving the strength and function of the connective tissue, collagen and elastin. As a result it really does help avoid wrinkles.
- If you notice a loss of elasticity in your skin, you need more silica in your diet.
- It is through the connective tissue that nutrients are absorbed and toxins excreted. By improving this function, silica gives skin greater vitality and means it absorbs skin products better.
- In addition, silica holds moisture, plumps and smoothes which means skin is better hydrated.
- Silica levels are highest just before birth and they decline with each passing year as the body ages.
- RDA is unknown.

Best food sources:
Whole grains, oats, barley, millet, onions, beetroot, potatoes, horsetail herb.

Zinc

This is another important immune booster – you will most likely have seen it added to some cold remedies. It increases the production of T cells – the white blood cells produced by the thymus gland which are important in fighting infection. See page 35 for more about zinc's antioxidant properties.

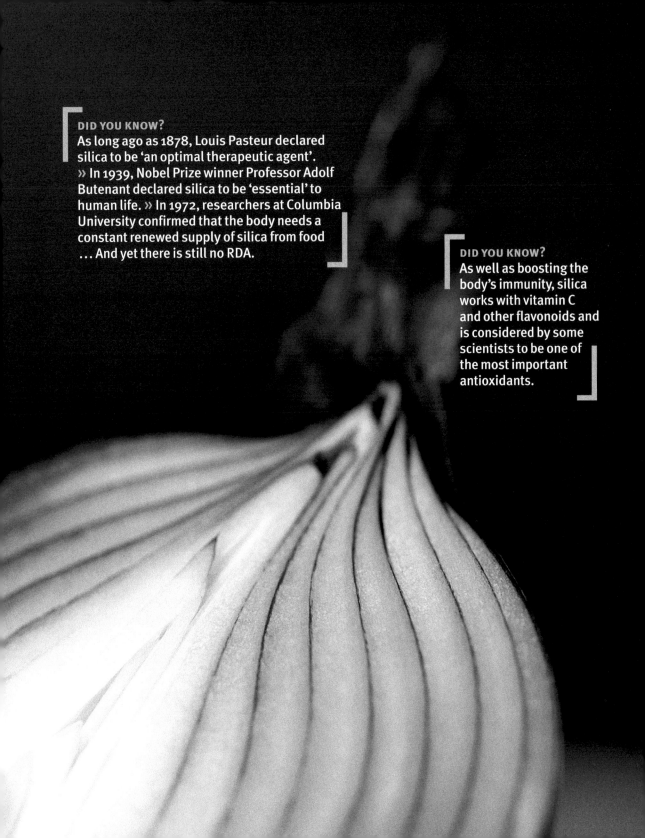

DID YOU KNOW?
As long ago as 1878, Louis Pasteur declared silica to be 'an optimal therapeutic agent'. » In 1939, Nobel Prize winner Professor Adolf Butenant declared silica to be 'essential' to human life. » In 1972, researchers at Columbia University confirmed that the body needs a constant renewed supply of silica from food … And yet there is still no RDA.

DID YOU KNOW?
As well as boosting the body's immunity, silica works with vitamin C and other flavonoids and is considered by some scientists to be one of the most important antioxidants.

Essential fatty acids

It is impossible to miss the hype about essential fatty acids or EFAs. They are the 'good' fats we all need and much heralded in news stories, magazines and healthy eating plans. They are particularly found in nuts, seeds, fish oils and oily fish like salmon. And they really do live up to their reputation as super nutrients. They offer vital anti-inflammatory protection and stimulate and support the immune system as well as providing amazing antioxidant protection.

Good fat facts

···} Essential fatty acids are defined as fats which are essential to human health but cannot actually be manufactured by the body. This means they have to be obtained through diet.

···} Scientists describe EFAs as long-chain polyunsaturated fatty acids which are derived from linolenic (Omega-3), linoleic (Omega-6) and oleic (Omega-9) acids.

···} Omega-9 is necessary but is not strictly speaking an essential fatty acid as the body can produce a small amount itself.

···} Skin cell membranes are themselves composed of essential fats.

···} By eating EFAs we are protecting cell membranes and the lipid layers that surround vital areas of the cell, inflammation is kept to a minimum, cells are not stressed and signs of ageing are slowed.

···} Essential fatty acids help stabilize skin cells and prevent the formation of inflammatory chemicals including arachidonic acid, one of the prime causes of inflammation.

···} A lack of essential fats will cause cells to dry out too quickly, resulting in dry skin and an excessive need for moisturizers.

···} This deficiency will leave skin looking obviously dry and dehydrated and will speed the formation of lines and wrinkles.

Omega acids

···> A healthy diet is dependent upon maintaining the correct balance between Omega-3 and Omega-6 fatty acids. Omega-3 is mainly found in fish and plant oils while Omega-6 is more common in meat and dairy products, although it is also found in evening primrose oil and borage oil. Dieticians believe the optimum balance between the two is about twice as much Omega-6 as Omega-3.

···> The modern (US-type diet) is much more likely to contain high levels of Omega-6 than Omega-3, which causes problems as too high a level of Omega-6 suppresses the absorption of Omega-3. Omega-3 is also needed for the body to properly utilize Omega-6 fatty acids.

···> To improve Omega-3 levels, experts recommend we adopt a more Mediterranean-style diet, basically comprising more fish (especially oily cold water fish like salmon, mackerel, sardines, anchovies and herring), along with plenty of fresh fruit and vegetables, garlic, onions, whole grains and olive oil. Meat plays a much less important role in this type of diet than in, say, a typical American one.

DID YOU KNOW?

High levels of salt, processed food, saturated fat and trans fatty acids, as well as pollution, smoking, stress and alcohol, all work to stop the body making good use of essential fatty acids.

DID YOU KNOW?

An average US diet typically consists of between 11 and 30 times more Omega-6 than Omega-3 fatty acids. There is a growing belief among researchers that this is a prime cause of the rising rates of inflammatory disorders. » A lack of essential fatty acids can lead to a variety of health problems including weight gain, depression, skin problems and accelerated ageing as your body simply won't be able to maintain normal bodily functions.

Omega-3 facts

There are three major types which are used by the body:

⋯⇒ ALA (alpha-linolenic acid)

⋯⇒ EPA (eicosapentaenoic acid)

⋯⇒ DHA (docosahexaenoic acid)

⋯⇒ Extensive studies have shown that as well as reducing inflammation, Omega-3 fatty acids help prevent heart disease, diabetes and arthritis and improve brain function, as well as controlling insulin levels and excess weight.

⋯⇒ Omega-3 fatty acids are used in the formation of cell walls, making them supple and flexible and improving oxygen uptake and circulation.

⋯⇒ Omega-3s are particularly efficient at targeting the compounds which cause allergic reactions and skin disorders.

⋯⇒ Studies show that Omega-3 reduces the itching and scaliness which is associated with psoriasis.

⋯⇒ Omega-3 fatty acids are more likely to be damaged in cooking and processing than Omega-6.

⋯⇒ The Omega-3 found in vegetable sources such as soya and flax oils have to be converted to DHA and EPA by the body, whereas the majority of Omega-3 in fish and fish oils is already in that form.

Best food sources:
Cold water fish (including salmon, mackerel, sardines, anchovies, herring, tuna), walnuts, pumpkin seeds, flaxseeds and oil, soya, cold-pressed canola oil, avocados and leafy green vegetables. Always look for unprocessed, unrefined oils to ensure optimum supplies of Omega-3.

DID YOU KNOW?
Hemp oil is a good vegetarian source of Omega-3 if you don't eat fish. It is also rich in antioxidant vitamin E and helps preserve young-looking skin. It contains more EFAs than flaxseed oil and has a pleasant, nutty taste. There's also no danger of getting high on it – the cannabinoid levels are way too low. It should not be heated, however, as cooking breaks down the omega fats.

'You can't help getting older, but you don't have to get old.'

GEORGE BURNS

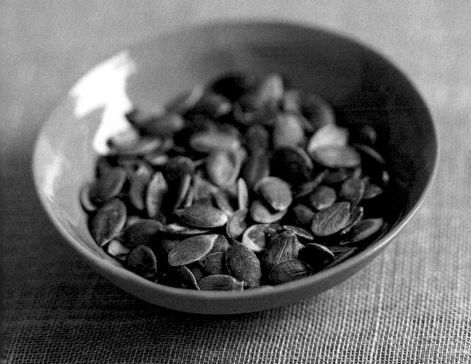

DID YOU KNOW?
Clinicians have shown that flaxseeds which are high in Omega-3 can help in the treatment of acne.

DID YOU KNOW?
Initial studies suggest that omega fatty acids may help reduce sun sensitivity.

Omega-6 facts

···⟩ Linoleic acid is the major Omega-6 fatty acid. In healthy bodies with good balanced diets this is converted into gamma linolenic acid (GLA).

···⟩ GLA is then synthesized with EPA from the Omega-3 group into DGLA and then into prostaglandins, which are hormone-like substances.

···⟩ These prostaglandins are essential for normal body functions and, among other things, prevent blood clots, lower blood pressure, maintain water balance, decrease inflammation and pain, improve immune function and help insulin to work.

···⟩ Omega-6 acids can help skin disorders like psoriasis and eczema.

···⟩ A diet which is too high in Omega-6 inhibits the absorption of Omega-3.

Best food sources:
Evening primrose oil and borage oil are the best sources of GLA; flaxseeds and oil, hempseed, grapeseed oil, pumpkin seeds, sunflower seeds, blackcurrant seed oil, pistachios, pine nuts, olives and olive oil, and chicken.

'I think your whole life shows in your face and you should be proud of that.' LAUREN BACALL

Omega-9 facts

···> Although essential for health, it is
technically not an essential fatty acid
because the body can manufacture small
amounts itself provided other EFAs are
present in the diet.

···> It is a monounsaturated fatty acid.

···> Also known as oleic acid.

···> It is used by the body to fight inflammation,
prevent the build up of fatty deposits in
the arteries, maintain the blood sugar
balance and improve the functioning of
the immune system.

···> Essential fatty acids are also crucial for
the healthy functioning of nerve cells
in the brain.

Best food sources:
Olives and olive oil, fruit and, in particular,
berries, peanuts and avocados.

EAT YOUR FISH AND STOP FACIAL SAGGING
As well as being the best source of omega fatty acids, fish also contain a chemical
compound called dimethylaminoethanol, or DMAE. This is a neurotransmitter which
is found in small amounts in the human brain and research shows it can actually halt
and even reverse facial sagging. » DMAE basically stimulates the production of another
neurotransmitter called acetylcholine which works to stabilize cell membranes. It is
also a powerful antioxidant preventing free radical damage but the great news for skin
is that it improves skin tone, increasing firmness by stimulating muscles and nerves,
stopping the signs of ageing. The best source of DMAE is wild, cold-water salmon.

Blood sugar and skin

Blood sugar or blood glucose levels are fundamentally important to how our bodies work as glucose is the basic fuel for the central nervous system.

⋯⇢ If blood levels fall too low for a significant period of time you can fall into a coma and eventually die.

⋯⇢ High sugar levels in diabetics are associated with a range of serious problems including heart disease, kidney failure and blindness.

⋯⇢ It is probably less well known that blood sugar levels can also have a dramatic effect on the skin and can actually speed up the ageing process, causing wrinkles.

DID YOU KNOW?
Cinnamon can help control blood sugar levels and has been used in the treatment of type-2 diabetes. A 2003 study in the journal *Diabetes Care* suggested that 1-6g of the spice a day 'significantly reduced blood-sugar levels'.

DID YOU KNOW?
Diabetics whose blood sugar levels are not adequately controlled age a third faster than non-diabetics.

The problem:

⋯⇢ As well as being an essential fuel, glucose can damage cells and tissues causing cellular inflammation throughout the body.

⋯⇢ High blood sugar levels trigger a number of chemical reactions. These result in the creation of free radicals which attack cell membranes. In turn this releases inflammatory chemicals which create more damage and accelerate ageing.

⋯⇢ This process is known as glycation and one of the most serious results is cross-linking, which is the formation of chemical bridges between proteins and other large molecules.

⋯⇢ Anything that undergoes this process generally becomes harder, loses elasticity and is easily damaged.

⋯⇢ In our bodies, cross-linking causes joints to stiffen and arteries to harden.

⋯⇢ In the skin, cross-linking causes collagen to lose its elasticity and flexibility. Lines created naturally through facial expressions stop smoothing out and become fixed wrinkles which deepen into folds.

The anti-ageing solution:

---> The rate at which carbohydrates in food are broken down into sugars is measured by the glycaemic index. Foods which break down quickly are high-glycaemic and cause a surge in insulin levels as the body struggles to control the level of blood sugar.

---> To stay young, the answer is to choose foods with a low-glycaemic index. These take longer to break down and are absorbed more gradually, meaning that the body does not have to deal with rapid rises in sugars and insulin levels remain healthily steady. Another positive side-effect is that you will feel satisfied for longer and so are less likely to snack unhealthily and put on extra weight.

---> Low-glycaemic food sources include: fruits, vegetables, oats and whole grains, nuts, lentils, soya and olive oil, plus good sources of protein such as fish and chicken. For more information see page 84.

DID YOU KNOW?
Whole grain rye bread has a 32 per cent lower glycaemic rating than white bread. No prizes for guessing which is better for you!

'Alas, after a certain age every man is responsible for his face.'

ALBERT CAMUS

Changes to hormone levels

As we age, most hormone levels decline, in particular the so-called youth hormones, oestrogen and human growth hormone. A lack of the latter in particular affects muscle tone, weakens connective tissue and results in a loss of skin thickness, firmness and suppleness. It is human growth hormone, or HGH, which is responsible for the smooth appearance of children's skin. Clinical studies have shown that skin cells treated with HGH grow evenly, reproducing the smooth texture of youth.

- The slowing down of the hormonal system is an important part of the ageing process – particularly the functioning of the thyroid and adrenal glands.
- Human growth hormone, or HGH, is produced in the pituitary gland, a tiny gland at the base of the brain.
- The pituitary gland regulates the entire hormone system.
- The only hormone to increase as we age is cortisol, the stress hormone.
- Although cortisol is essential to overcome stress, large amounts can be harmful over long periods of time.
- Cortisol is associated with old age and, along with other effects, it can deplete the immune system and cause skin to thin.
- High cortisol levels also cause a rise in blood sugar and insulin levels.

Boosting youth hormones

There are no foods which we can eat to supply us with human growth hormone, but there are some simple steps you can take to boost your body's production of the hormone.

The most important factor is making sure you get sufficient sleep. This is when growth hormone is released and when the bad effects of too much cortisol are overcome.

To help sleep:

- Avoid caffeine from mid-afternoon.
- Don't eat too late – there should be at least two hours between your last meal and bedtime.
- Choose low glycaemic foods and avoid anything which will cause a rush of sugars and insulin.
- Opt for foods high in complex carbohydrates and proteins rather than simple sugars.
- Avoid alcohol just before bed. Although it can initially make you feel sleepy, too much often prompts you to wake around 3am.

DID YOU KNOW?
Too much alcohol results in red thread veins and broken capillaries in the skin.

DID YOU KNOW?
Salt and processed food can cause water retention, leaving skin looking puffy.

DID YOU KNOW?
According to a study in the US, women who drink at least two 250ml (8fl oz) servings of skimmed milk a day are 44 per cent more likely to develop acne. Scientists think this may be due to hormones in the milk. Research suggests that soya and soya products may actually reduce acne.

And finally . . . drink water!

It's such an obvious thing to do and yet many people simply don't drink enough. And no, you can't get away with substituting tea, coffee or fruit juice – in fact, for every cup of coffee you drink, you should also sip a glass of water to compensate for the diuretic effect of the coffee.

I always start the day with a mug of warm water and a slice of lemon. I find it really wakes me up and I know it's doing me good. The warm water helps to remove ageing toxins and the lemon improves my skin's elasticity. I stand by my assertion that water is the body's most fundamental beauty treatment. Without sufficient water we simply dry up.

···} The average adult is 60–70 per cent water and although we can last several weeks without food, we can survive only a few days without water. Water is essential for the body to function properly – it hydrates cells, washes away waste and carries nutrients through the blood. If you're not drinking enough your body may even retain water to try to compensate. And don't wait to feel thirsty – the thirst mechanism actually declines with age.

···} Nutritionists recommend drinking between eight and ten glasses of water a day, which is roughly 2 litres (4½ pints), and if you are exercising or it is very hot, you may well need more.

···} The good news is that the benefits of drinking water quickly become obvious when you look in the mirror. Your skin will appear clearer and less puffy, it will feel noticeably softer and fine lines will be less obvious.

My top tips for youthful, healthy skin

···➤ You may not be able to alter the hand nature and your genes have dealt you but you can make the most of it.

···➤ Eat a variety of foods, especially fresh fruits and vegetables.

···➤ Each is unique and by eating foods in combination with one another you are doing as much as you can to ensure optimum absorption of vital vitamins, minerals and other nutrients.

···➤ Choose fruit and vegetables from the red-purple-orange colour spectrum to maximize your intake of free-radical attacking antioxidants.

···➤ Leafy greens like spinach and broccoli are also antioxidant-rich as well as providing vitamins A, C and E.

···➤ Don't forget protein, especially oily fish like salmon which are packed full of essential youth-preserving omega fatty acids.

···➤ Protein and slow-release carbohydrates will ensure a steady flow of insulin and protect you from damaging surges in blood sugar levels.

···➤ Snacking on nuts and seeds keeps you going (without resorting to sugary carbohydrates) and adds amazing minerals and essential fatty acids to your diet.

···➤ Keep skin well hydrated by drinking lots and lots of water.

'Old age is no place for sissies.'
BETTE DAVIS

Body food

Youth is associated with health and vitality and while we all like the idea of looking young, it is equally important, and perhaps more so, to actually feel young. Bodily ageing is much more to do with what's going on inside and general health. Nothing is more ageing than stiff limbs, a lack of energy and the age-related illnesses which are made worse and often caused by a poor diet.

By balancing the food you eat, making sure it contains plenty of good things and limits the bad, you will feel and look younger and healthier. I'm not a fan of diets, so I'm not talking about dieting here or constantly worrying about what you eat. But armed with a little knowledge and a few adjustments, you can still enjoy mealtimes, feel satisfied and know you're doing yourself good. You will be more energetic, sleep better, look more toned and will be protecting your body from a range of diseases. You may even find you lose a few pounds along the way.

DID YOU KNOW?
According to the American Institute for Cancer Research, around 40 per cent of cancers are diet related. Eating at least five portions of fruit and vegetables each day cuts the risk of breast, lung, bowel and bladder cancers.

The ageing body

Bone density

As we age, our bone mineral density (or BMD) falls. BMD is essentially a measure of the amount of calcified tissue within our bones and is a guide to how strong they are.

A loss of bone density is a normal part of ageing for both women and men, typically beginning between the ages of 30 and 40. Studies have shown that in women the menopause is followed by an increased rate of bone loss which usually continues for about ten years, after which the rate of loss slows again.

All the bones in our bodies are composed of a thick outer wall and a strong inner mesh which is made up of collagen, calcium salts and other minerals. Problems arise when this inner mesh weakens to such a degree that the spaces become bigger, leaving bones fragile and more easily broken – a process called osteoporosis.

The rate of bone density loss

There are two parts to bone structure which are called cortical and trabecular. Cortical bone is the hard outer shell and makes up 75 per cent of total bone mass. Trabecular bone is the spongy interior mesh of bones and so makes up most of the bone volume. Bone is a highly active tissue, which is constantly being remodelled with a balance between new bone forming and the resorption of old bone.

- Bone density peaks around the age of 30 for both men and women.
- After this age, roughly 0.4 per cent of bone mass is lost each year.
- This rate continues steadily for healthy men and women until women reach the menopause, at which point the rate accelerates.
- The average rate of loss for healthy, postmenopausal women is between 1 and 2 per cent.
- The rate of loss can vary throughout the body.
- In the first five to ten years after menopause, rates of loss are usually higher – between 2 and 4 per cent.

Osteoporosis

Osteoporosis means porous bones. It's estimated that osteoporosis affects 3 million people in the UK. In the US it affects 25 million people and half of all women over 45. Each year there are over 230,000 fractures as a result of the condition.

Factors which increase the risk of osteoporosis include:

⋯⋗ A lack of oestrogen for women and testosterone for men.

⋯⋗ Early menopause – before the age of 45.

⋯⋗ Missing periods for over six months as a result of over-dieting or excessive exercise.

⋯⋗ Family history of the disease.

⋯⋗ Malabsorption of nutrients – through conditions like coeliac disease or Crohn's disease.

⋯⋗ Studies show a lack of calcium in the diet has a significant effect on bone loss in women. If the body does not receive enough calcium, it will begin to take it from the bones.

⋯⋗ It is important to make sure your diet supplies enough calcium throughout your life, ideally from childhood, long before problems like osteoporosis become apparent.

⋯⋗ Heavy drinking deprives the body of vital nutrients especially calcium and vitamin D. It also interferes with normal healthy bone turnover.

⋯⋗ Smoking also depletes vitamins and minerals and can lead to an earlier menopause and breakdown of oestrogen.

What you can do to help

⋯⋗ Eat a healthy well balanced diet, with a range of foods from each of the different food groups, including protein, vitamins and minerals. Bone mineral loss begins long before there are any outward signs.

⋯⋗ Boost calcium and vitamin D levels and the natural production of hormones through diet. Supplements of calcium, vitamin D and bisphosphonates (as prescribed by a GP) may also help bone density and reduce the likelihood of fractures.

⋯⋗ Make sure you take regular exercise. Weight-bearing exercise, walking, tennis and yoga are all particularly helpful.

DID YOU KNOW?
The skeleton takes just two years to completely renew itself in childhood. An adult skeleton takes between seven and ten years.

> **DID YOU KNOW?**
> Eating an orange with your meal means you will absorb more calcium, iron, minerals and other vitamins from your food.

Body building – calcium

Calcium plays a vital role in the formation of bones and their maintenance. The Scientific Advisory Committee on Nutrition which sets recommended daily levels for nutrient consumption advises that calcium intake should be over 700mg daily for an adult. However, many scientists think this should be higher and set at an optimum level of around 1000mg and as much as 1200mg during pregnancy and breastfeeding. Ideally, for healthily strong bones and to guard against osteoporosis later in life, you should eat a calcium-rich diet from childhood.

It is worth remembering that for calcium to be properly absorbed, your body also needs vitamin D. Obviously if you play a sport outdoors or take regular walks, sunlight will help you to make your own vitamin D. The best food source of the vitamin is oily fish.

> **DID YOU KNOW?**
> 'Calcium is essential for healthy bones but also plays a fundamental role in maintaining the normal structure of the skin,' says Professor Peter Elias, University of California. This is because calcium is essential for the absorption of nutrients through cell membranes.

Useful facts

- Dairy products contain the most easily absorbed calcium, although there is very little in either butter or cream.
- Some common foods can radically reduce calcium absorption. These include wholegrain cereals, bran and some nuts and pulses which contain phytic acid (a naturally-occurring compound found in cereals and legumes). This means that a 250ml (8fl oz) serving of milk on your wholegrain breakfast cereal will supply a tiny fraction of the calcium that the same serving would provide if drunk as a plain glass of milk at a different time of day.
- The oxalic acid in vegetables like spinach and some greens can also reduce calcium absorption.
- Coca-cola and other fizzy drinks contain phosphoric acid which increases the amount of calcium your body loses.

Good food sources of calcium include:
Dairy products, bony fish (especially sardines and whitebait), tofu, sesame seeds, almonds, dried figs, watercress, parsley and okra.

Muscle loss

Just as bone density reaches a peak and then begins to decline with age, muscles begin to lose mass from the early 30s onwards. In 1988 Dr I Rosenberg, from the Human Nutrition Research Center on Ageing at Tufts University, Boston, identified this process as 'sarcopenia' which literally means 'vanishing flesh' and medically refers to the loss of skeletal muscle mass.

It is estimated that skeletal muscle mass decreases between 35 and 40 per cent on average between the ages of 20 and 80 for both men and women.

Even though someone may weigh the same at 50 as they did at 30, they are likely to have lost muscle.

This loss is often hidden as the body simply replaces muscle with fat.

Muscle loss dramatically increases at menopause. Some researchers believe the increase is as much as six times the normal rate and have linked it with the loss of oestrogen.

The loss of muscle mass has important implications for our bodies as it leads to weakness which makes falls more likely and can make any problems with thinning bones much worse.

What you can do to help

Vitamin E

Tufts University Human Nutrition Research Center on Ageing found that vitamin E substantially reduces muscle and free radical damage to muscles after exercise.

Hormones

Studies suggest that testosterone supplementation may slow age-related muscle loss in men.

Results of studies showed testosterone supplements increased fat-free body mass as well as muscle size and strength.

Human Growth Hormone has also been heralded as a potential 'fountain of youth'.

A study published in the New England Journal of Medicine reported significant increases in muscle mass and bone density in men after taking HGH.

Subsequent studies, mainly carried out in the US, have shown that HGH supplements restore youthful levels of the hormone in women and can also improve skeletal muscle mass.

It is hard not to be impressed by the anti-ageing possibilities of HGH but there are side effects, including headaches, water retention and swelling joints.

Supplements

···≯ Creatine, which is found in meat, poultry and fish, boosts the amount of ATP (adenosine tri-phosphate) which is a high energy phosphate molecule used by muscles for short bursts of power.

···≯ Researchers have described creatine as acting like car fuel, powering skeletal muscle cells.

···≯ Clinical studies have shown that creatine increases muscle strength and power in middle-aged men.

···≯ Carnosine is a natural compound which is made up of amino acids and is found in high concentrations in skeletal muscles.

···≯ Levels of carnosine fall by 63 per cent in our bodies between the ages of 10 and 70.

···≯ Anti-ageing researchers are very excited by test results which suggest that carnosine supplements may halt the development of sarcopenia – skeletal muscle loss.

···≯ Carnosine is a powerful free-radical scavenger and it is thought it is this quality which gives its anti-ageing effect.

···≯ The best food sources of carnosine are meat, poultry and fish which are all complete proteins.

Amino acids

···≯ Amino acid supplements may prompt the body to produce its own HGH without the side-effects or cost of HGH supplements.

···≯ An initial study in 1981 repeated more recently in 1997, showed that two amino acids, l-arginine and l-lysine, increased HGH levels when taken together.

···≯ Relatively low doses of 1500mg of each were prescribed and, interestingly, HGH levels only increased when the two were taken together. If taken separately there was no effect.

In addition, for healthy, supple bones and muscles it's essential to make sure your diet is supplying an adequate amount of good-quality protein.

Body-building protein

Protein is absolutely essential for building every cell in the body. Muscles, bones, tissues (including collagen), organs, enzymes for digestion and the antibodies which protect against infection are all made of protein. All our cells are composed of amino acids and when proteins are digested they are broken down into amino acids, which cells use to repair themselves. Put simply, protein is vital for cellular repair and rebuilding and without it, the ageing process is accelerated.

Recommended daily amounts vary, but dieticians recommend at least 65g for women and 75g for men. To put this in perspective, an average portion of lean chicken would supply around 28g of protein.

Best food sources:

Fish, meat and animal sources of protein (including eggs and dairy products) usually provide a complete protein in themselves, whereas you would need to eat a combination of vegetables including pulses, legumes like peas and beans, and cereals to obtain a complete vegetable source of protein (the only exception to this is soya). The downside to many meats is the high level of saturated fat they also contain. For this reason dieticians tend to recommend lean poultry, game, fish and low-fat dairy products.

DID YOU KNOW?
Our bodies cannot store protein and so it must be supplied daily through the food we eat. » If you eat too much protein, the excess is converted into fats and sugars.

Cellulite

This isn't just a problem associated with weight. Many otherwise slim women are plagued by that all-too familiar dimpled effect everyone hates. You've only got to flick through the summer editions of celebrity magazines to see photos of svelte celebs caught off guard with, horror of horrors, orange-peel thighs, proving they too are only human.

As we saw earlier in this chapter (see page 32), progressive damage by free radicals leads to a loss of collagen and elastin, together with hyaluronic acid which helps keep the dermis hydrated. Skin loses its bounce and resilience and can no longer smooth over the subcutaneous fat layer below. This means fat cells show through, giving the characteristic dimpled effect of cellulite.

Scientists now think there is a link between a poor blood supply to the fat cells and the build-up of fluid and other toxins which cause cellulite to develop. Improving the quality of the food you eat rather than simply looking at the quantity can help.

'Cellulite is not a problem of too much fat. Rather, it is a problem of too little water.'

DR HOWARD MURAD, LEADING DERMATOLOGIST AND SKINCARE EXPERT

Cellulite-promoting foods to avoid:

····⟫ Caffeine – too much causes blood vessels to constrict and affects circulation.

····⟫ Salt – high levels make skin puffy and lead to water retention which can emphasize the appearance of cellulite. It's worth remembering that many packaged foods contain high levels of hidden salt.

····⟫ Saturated fat, sugar, processed foods, starchy foods, alcohol, stress and smoking all generate toxins which trigger free radicals and put pressure on the lymph system. A sluggish lymph system does not drain toxins adequately and actually creates fibres which bind to the walls of fat cells, making them even thicker.

Banish cellulite by eating more:

····⟫ Lean protein which is vital for healthy growth and cell repair. Poultry or fish are ideal.

····⟫ Fruit and vegetables, especially the brightly coloured ones which are packed with antioxidant flavonoids. These will boost collagen and keep skin supple and smooth.

····⟫ Essential fatty acids, especially Omega-3 rich salmon. This will help balance cholesterol levels and so boost circulation. EFAs are also important to maintain healthy, pliable cell walls.

Good cellulite-fighting foods include: pomegranates, apples, kelp, fennel, oranges, rosemary, ginger, garlic, cayenne, cinnamon, pepper, cloves, onions, whole grains, raw fruit and vegetables.

DID YOU KNOW?
Dehydration speeds up ageing. And you can't use thirst as a guide because your thirst mechanism functions less effectively as you age.

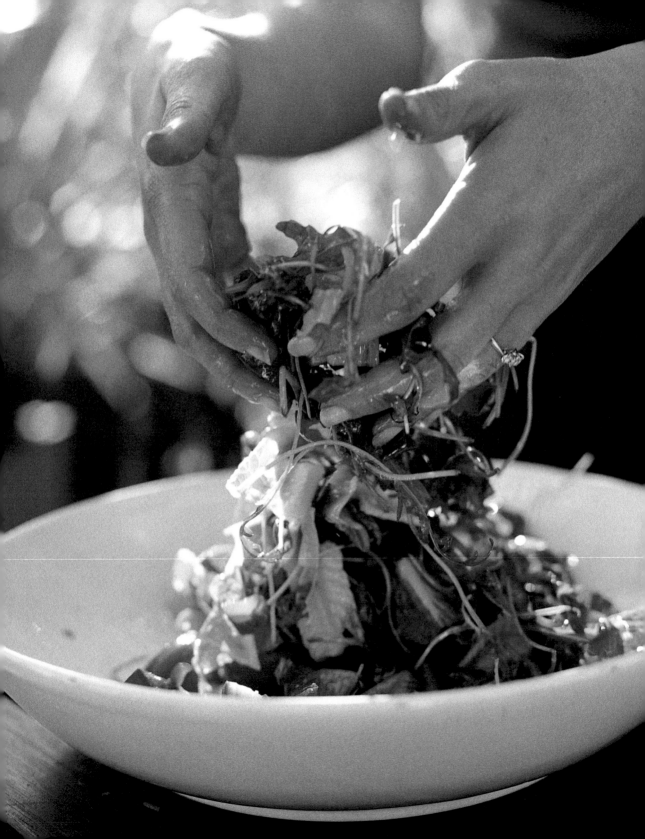

Drink more water

Studies show that areas of cellulite contain higher than average numbers of water-retaining cells. Excess fluid gravitates towards these, causing them to swell. This is a major cause of cellulite in thinner women.

···› Not drinking enough water can actually make the problem of water retention worse as the body believes it is dehydrated and must conserve every tiny amount.

···› Nutritionists recommend drinking between eight and ten glasses a day, which is around 2 litres (4½ pints).

···› Don't forget water-rich foods like cucumbers and salad leaves, which can boost your fluid intake if you find drinking enough water a struggle.

···› As an alternative, try supplementing your water intake with green tea – it is a good antioxidant as well as helping you stay hydrated.

DID YOU KNOW?
Apples are full of the fibre pectin, making them an ideal fruit for combating cellulite. Pectin also helps reduce cholesterol levels. » Pomegranates are another excellent weapon. They contain ellagic acid which strengthens blood vessels and protects cells. » A low-fibre diet makes cellulite worse.

DID YOU KNOW?
Cucumbers are 80 per cent water and a good source of vitamin C. Don't peel the skin – it's rich in fibre and silica, an essential component of healthy tissue.

Weight matters

I'm going to say straight off that I don't believe in dieting. The philosophy is short term, hence results don't last and they don't encourage you to change the way you eat on a daily basis. But I am in favour of healthy eating. And by this I don't mean boring, or measly portions with a long list of banned ingredients.

Choosing the right foods will ensure an adequate supply of antioxidants vital for combating the ageing attacks of free radicals. It will also boost immunity and protect you from diseases like cancer, heart disease and diabetes – all of which become more common as we age. I have seen so many people completely transformed by just a few changes to their diets. There are still a lot of misconceptions around about food, but armed with some key facts it's possible to find out what's right for you in terms of both what you eat and how you eat. I promise you will be trimmed, toned and, most importantly, healthy after just a few weeks, looking and feeling years younger.

Your metabolic rate slows and your body burns calories between 2 and 4 per cent more slowly with each passing decade. No matter what shape you started out, from your 30s onwards any extra weight tends to head for the hips and waist and stays put. Sadly, middle-aged spread isn't a myth and there's no doubt that extra weight is ageing.

DID YOU KNOW?
It is better to drink water at room temperature or even warm. Cold water chills your stomach and means it absorbs nutrients less efficiently.

Your metabolic rate

---> Metabolism is the process of converting food either into energy, to be used for bodily repairs, or to be stored as fat for future use.

---> The rate at which this process happens varies considerably.

---> People with a faster metabolism burn calories more efficiently and store less fat.

---> Those with a slower metabolic rate burn calories less efficiently and, as a consequence, more calories are stored as fat.

---> Overweight people tend to have a slower metabolic rate than slim people.

---> Resting metabolic rate, or basal metabolic rate, is the number of calories needed to maintain essential bodily processes. This usually accounts for 60 per cent of all the calories eaten.

---> The heavier a person is, the more calories are needed to fuel these essential functions.

DID YOU KNOW?

In 2005 a British Parliamentary committee found that two-thirds of the country's population were overweight or obese, which represents a four-fold increase in the past 25 years. Problems associated with this are now costing up to £7.4 billion per year.

DID YOU KNOW?

Overeating is one of the main causes of ageing and increases the risk of heart disease and many cancers. The British Heart Foundation figures show that coronary heart disease causes 270,000 deaths a year and attributes 28,000 of these to obesity.

Our personal metabolic rate is determined by a number of factors:

Age – our calorie needs decrease typically by 2 per cent each decade as our metabolic rate slows.

Genes – some people are born with a naturally faster metabolism. Sadly it really is true that while some people can apparently eat whatever they want with no obvious effect, others seem to put on weight if they so much as look at a chocolate bar.

How often we eat – our metabolic rate increases while we are digesting food. This process is called the thermal effect of food and is the reason why some people feel noticeably warmer after eating. In fact, research suggests the metabolic rate rises by 20 to 30 per cent every time we eat and remains high for the next couple of hours. This is very important as it means that if we go too long without eating, our metabolism misses out on this boost. Also our body is fooled into thinking there is a food shortage and our metabolic rate slows down accordingly to conserve energy. Typically, men can last five hours without eating but women should go no longer than three hours if they don't want to affect their metabolism.

Muscle to fat body ratio – muscle cells need about eight times more energy to sustain them than fat cells, which means that the higher our proportion of muscle to fat, the faster our metabolic rate.

How active we are – it's obvious, but exercise burns more calories than sitting still. And the effect keeps on going. Even after we stop exercising the body continues to burn calories at a faster rate for several hours.

Nutrition – to metabolize food efficiently, our body has to perform thousands of chemical reactions. For these to happen, we need a range of nutrients and particularly vitamin C and vitamins B2, B3, B5 and B6. A balanced, varied diet is the best way to ensure good dietary nutrition.

DIET PILLS
Can fat-burning pills or supplements actually speed up metabolism and help weight loss? The answer is a simple and unequivocal no. Dieticians do not consider this a safe method of raising the metabolism and nor has it been proved to help long-term weight loss.

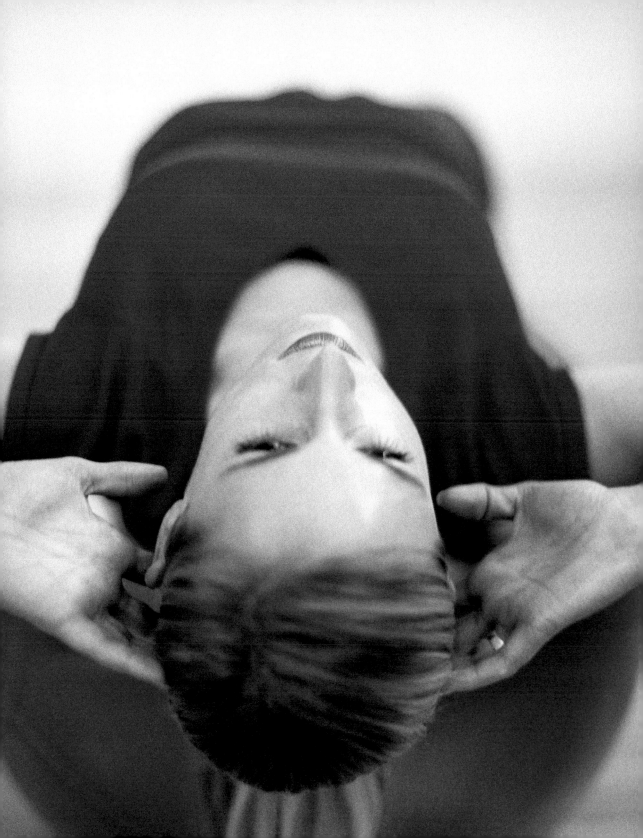

How to raise your metabolic rate safely

···> The first step is to eat a balanced diet, supplying your body with all the nutrients, vitamins and minerals it needs to keep your metabolism running efficiently.

···> Eat breakfast. This really is the most important meal of the day. Your metabolic rate slows by 5 per cent overnight and stays at this level until you next eat. For healthy breakfast choices, see page 240.

···> Take regular exercise, especially anything that raises the heart rate and those which help to build and maintain muscle.

Several foods and drinks appear to raise the metabolic rate:

···> Chilli and other hot spices lead to an increased heart rate for up to three hours after eating.

···> Protein has a higher thermal effect, burning more calories during digestion, but high-protein diets can also mean high levels of saturated fat and have been linked with the loss of bone calcium and kidney problems.

···> Caffeine drinks increase heart rate and metabolism, while green tea increases metabolism without affecting the heart rate.
Note: The over-consumption of any of these foods for weight loss is not recommended as there may be side effects which could damage your health.

FAT HORMONES AND METABOLISM
Recent research at the University of Pennsylvania Medical Center has highlighted a hormone called adiponectin, found in fat tissue, which, it appears, may boost metabolism and cause weight loss without affecting the appetite. This follows the earlier discovery of leptin, another fat hormone, which encourages weight loss and raises the metabolism by suppressing the appetite. » This may have implications for the future as this hormone could overcome the problem of weight loss becoming more difficult as the body compensates for lowered calorie intake by slowing the metabolic rate. Dr Rexford Ahima, Assistant Professor of Medicine at the University of Pennsylvania, says, 'Adiponectin or its targets in the brain and other organs could be harnessed to sustain weight loss by maintaining a high metabolic rate. This is only a possibility. We're not suggesting at this point that Adiponectin will become a drug.'

Why calorie-controlled diets often fail

How many people do you know who have diligently followed a strict calorie-controlled diet, lost the extra pounds, only to find that a few months later they are back to where they started or even more overweight? If you look at what happens to the metabolic rate, it is simple to understand why this happens.

···⟩ With crash diets of below 1000 calories a day, the body sees the reduction in food as a threat and slows the metabolic rate by as much as 45 per cent.

···⟩ Once you've reached your ideal weight, you end up piling the pounds back on as soon as you go back to eating normally, because your metabolic rate has fallen so drastically and you now need less food to maintain a stable weight.

···⟩ This is why so many people end up dieting several times a year and not just once.

···⟩ Low-fat diets which cut out virtually all fat are especially doomed. You are depriving your body of an absolutely essential food and it is much more likely that you will feel hungry and unsatisfied. Your metabolic rate will plummet and you will be encouraging wrinkles and other signs of ageing. If you choose the right fats you can actually help healthy weight loss (see page 79).

DID YOU KNOW?
Yo-yo dieting is not only bad for the body, it also leads to a sluggish metabolism and speeds up signs of ageing, encouraging wrinkles and sagging as a response to the repeated build up and reduction of fat under the skin.

High-protein low-carbohydrate diets

High-protein diets encourage dieters to base their meals around meat, eggs and cheese and often restrict carbohydrates such as whole grains, cereals, fruits and vegetables. They work on the principle that the body needs protein.

These diets became popular because they were easy to follow, dieters didn't feel hungry and found they could achieve quick results in terms of weight loss. But this comes at a price.

The problems

⟶ The diets are very restrictive and often don't include the variety of foods needed to meet basic nutritional needs.

⟶ Essential fatty acids, vitamins, minerals and fibre may all be lacking and the restricted diet means the body may well not be able to absorb any nutrients there are adequately.

⟶ Without sufficient carbohydrates in the diet for energy the body is unable to burn fat.

⟶ Weight is initially lost because the body loses water. The extra protein raises the levels of uric acid and urea in the blood. These are toxic by-products of protein metabolism and the body gets rid of them by flushing water through the kidneys. However, this diuretic effect also increases the loss of essential minerals, including calcium from bones which can lead to osteoporosis.

⟶ Protein is a crucial part of a healthy diet but you can have too much of a good thing. The body can't use the excess, which is broken down into fats and sugars.

⟶ Ketones are formed which are released into the bloodstream. These suppress appetite and can cause nausea. They are formed when your diet does not include sufficient carbohydrates and are a sign of high blood sugar levels and insufficient insulin, which means the body cannot use the sugar for energy.

⋯⋗ One result is that metabolism falls, but there are other serious health implications.

⋯⋗ There is an increased risk of kidney stones and liver disease.

⋯⋗ If ketone levels are high enough they may build up in the blood and can eventually lead to coma and death.

⋯⋗ High-protein animal foods are often also high in saturated fats, which can lead to heart disease, strokes and diabetes as well as increasing the risk of cancer.

⋯⋗ In terms of ageing, high-protein diets are among the worst. They stress the body, deprive it of vital nutrients and increase inflammation, accelerating ageing in every cell inside the body and breaking down collagen in the skin, causing wrinkles and sagging.

'I don't diet because it messes up your metabolism. Instead, I eat three meals a day, particularly lots of fruit for breakfast.'

CLAUDIA SCHIFFER

Developing healthy habits

There are four simple steps everyone can take to healthier nutrition which will make you look younger. They will also give you greater control over how quickly you age and how susceptible you are to a range of diseases.

Food for life

1 Eat breakfast – it's the most important meal of the day.
2 Bring back good fats – they're essential for your body and for maintaining a healthy weight, but you have to choose the right ones.
3 Balance your blood sugar levels – this is the best anti-ageing strategy.
4 Variety is key – eating a wide range of foods ensures your body has all the right nutrients in the best combinations.

DID YOU KNOW?
69 per cent of young women in Britain regularly miss breakfast. Those who eat breakfast weigh 3.5kg (8lb) less on average than those who skip it.

Breakfast is best

Always, and I do mean always, eat breakfast. It's the single most important meal of the day and should never be missed. It kick-starts your metabolism and gives you the energy to face the day ahead. If you are in the habit of missing breakfast, not only will you be slowing down your metabolism, you will also weaken your stomach and hamper your digestive system.

⋯⟩ If you skip breakfast you're more likely to crave unhealthy snacks and sugar. You'll be hit by an energy low later in the day as blood sugar levels dip and so eat more at lunch and dinner. This will mean extra calories that you won't actually use up and which will be stored as fat.

⋯⟩ Research shows people who don't eat breakfast are more likely to put on weight or be overweight.

⋯⟩ Skipping breakfast slows your metabolism – as your body has no food to supply energy it slows the metabolic rate to conserve energy.

⋯⟩ The lack of food can accelerate muscle loss as the body looks for energy elsewhere.

⋯⟩ Breakfast is a good opportunity to increase your fibre intake – important for health and weight (see page 86).

My favourite breakfast is a bowl of muesli, preferably with fresh fruit and live, natural yogurt. Oat-based wholegrain cereals are a particularly good choice, but for more ideas look at the 'Breakfast is best' food plan on page 239.

DID YOU KNOW?
A University of Nottingham study found that people who missed breakfast showed an increase in harmful LDL cholesterol levels and a tendency to over-eat snacks later. Eating breakfast keeps you slim and protects your heart at the same time.

Good fats vs bad fats

When I first trained as a dietician some years ago, the message was very much if you wanted to shed a few extra pounds you simply cut down on your fat consumption. Not so today. Our knowledge of the complex relationship between nutrition, health and the way our bodies behave has grown enormously in the last few years.

By simply cutting out all fat, you deprive your body of an essential nutrient, vital for the proper absorption of other foods. Your metabolic rate will fall, what you do eat won't satisfy you for long, you'll feel hungry all the time, and you're basically setting yourself up for failure. You'll also see the side-effects in a dull, dry, lifeless complexion, deeper wrinkles, a lack of energy and premature ageing.

Fat is a very important part of any healthy balanced diet – but it has to be the right type of fat.

⋯⟩ Research has shown that people following a vegan diet often lose weight. This is despite the fact that their diets were often high in both nutrients and calories due to a relatively high fat content. But... the crucial point seems to be that the fat came from nuts, seeds and their oils – it was not saturated animal fat.

⋯⟩ There is no need to add saturated fats to the diet.

⋯⟩ However, polyunsaturated fats and the essential fatty acids (EFAs) they contain are vital for health.

⋯⟩ Udo Erasmus, the American nutritionist and author of *Fats that Heal, Fats that Kill*, claims these essential fatty acids actually help burn fat.

⋯⟩ Reducing saturated fats in your diet and including nuts, seeds and oily fish achieves the best balance between a low saturated fat diet and essential nutrition.

DID YOU KNOW?
In a Californian experiment volunteers ate 70 almonds a day in conjunction with a calorie-controlled diet. On average their weight fell by 18 per cent. Testers attributed this to the fact that almonds are nutrient-dense, providing EFAs and healthy monounsaturated fat, protein and fibre, all of which contribute to feeling satisfied and full.

My top choices for healthy fats

Olive oil – this is a monounsaturated fat containing Omega-9. It helps your body absorb antioxidant vitamins A and E, boosts energy, keeps skin glowing and protects against heart disease. It may even guard against cancer. Always look for extra-virgin cold-pressed varieties as these have the highest nutritional value.
Ideal for: cooking (as it withstands heat) and salad dressings, also a delicious alternative to butter – try dipping fresh bread into extra virgin olive oil with a few drops of soy sauce or balsamic vinegar. If a recipe lists vegetable shortening in the ingredients, try replacing it with half the amount of olive oil plus a small pinch of salt.

Hemp seed oil – the balance of Omega-3 and -6 EFAs make this the perfect oil to lower cholesterol, boost the immune system and circulation, improve memory and help depression.
Ideal for: salad dressings, the nutty, slightly sweet taste make it a perfect alternative to olive oil. Cooking will destroy its EFAs.

Walnut oil – this is a good source of the antioxidant ellagic acid which tests have shown inhibits the growth of cancer cells. It also protects the skin from sun damage and reduces high cholesterol levels. Ideal for: adding to olive oil in salad dressings for a delicious walnut taste. It is unsuitable for frying, but can be used in place of other fats for baking.

Avocado oil – contains antioxidant carotenes and chlorophyll; it's also rich in vitamin E.
Ideal for: frying as it withstands high heat well because it has a high smoking point.

Sesame seed oil – a good source of vitamins B and E, minerals and trace elements like copper, calcium, iron and magnesium. Ideal for: adding flavour to stir fries just before serving and for mixing with olive oil in dressings. It burns easily and is unsuitable for cooking. Most supermarkets stock toasted sesame oil which has a good flavour but for high nutrient content, look out for untoasted varieties.

···⟩ **Flaxseed oil** – a good source of Omega-3 and Omega-6, with a slightly nutty flavour. Flax seeds are not easily digested and contain high levels of phytoestrogens. The oil is much lower in phytoestrogens, lowers blood pressure and calms digestive problems.
Ideal for: mixing with other oils as a dressing. Cooking will destroy the EFAs.

···⟩ **Pumpkin seed oil** – this is rich in vitamins A and E, zinc and EFAs.
Ideal for: adding flavour after cooking and for mixing with other oils in salad dressings. Again, high heats will destroy nutrients.

···⟩ **Canola oil** – this oil was developed in Canada as a cheaper alternative to olive oil. It is derived from rapeseed oil but has eliminated the chemical toxins which can make people ill after consuming too much rapeseed oil. It contains linolenic acid and vitamin E. As this is a relatively new oil, its long-term effects on health are not known. I include it here because it is useful for cooking, especially in a wok for stir fries.
Ideal for: cooking as it withstands heat well. It has little flavour.

···⟩ **Coconut oil** – for years this oil was not included on any 'healthy' list as it contains relatively high levels of saturated fat. But nutrition science never stands still. Coconut oil hit the news when it was alleged that Jennifer Aniston was eating it as part of the Coconut Diet which claims the oil can help weight loss. It contains high levels of medium chain triglycerides which some dieticians think boost the metabolism. There seems to be some proof that they may prevent weight gain though they may not prompt weight loss.
Ideal for: cooking, including frying at high temperatures.

⋯⟩ **Don't forget nuts and seeds:** walnuts, almonds, pine nuts, pistachios, pecans, cashews, hazelnuts, sesame, sunflower and pumpkin seeds all contain essential fatty acids as well as protein. Eating a combination will supply you with vitamins, minerals and a combination of Omegas-3, -6 and -9 and other EFAs.

Ideal for: snacking and sprinkling onto salads for added flavour and texture.

⋯⟩ **And finally, eat oily fish** – including salmon, tuna, sardines, mackerel, anchovies, whitebait and herring which all contain Omega-3. They are anti-inflammatory, guard against heart disease and are essential for the brain, central nervous system and healthy cell growth. They are also good sources of vitamin D and iodine for thyroid function. See page 160 for more about fish oil supplements.

Recommended: two to three portions of oily fish a week.

DID YOU KNOW?
With a few exceptions, EFAs are destroyed by high heat, light and oxygen, so when eating foods or oils for their EFAs opt for their raw form. For instance, raw nuts are a better source of nutrients than roasted and certain oils should never be used for cooking. No oil should ever be re-used. » When choosing oils, opt for the better quality, cold-pressed, extra-virgin varieties. These are less refined and processed, and therefore contain the highest levels of EFAs and nutrients. They should be in dark-coloured glass to protect them from light and should always be stored away from heat and sunlight. Nuts and seeds should not be kept for too long and may even benefit from being stored in the refrigerator.

DID YOU KNOW?
In the US peanut butter sales doubled in six months after researchers at Harvard announced that eating peanut butter is good for you and cuts your risk of developing diabetes.

Bad fat

Saturated fat – too much saturated fat in the diet can lead to raised cholesterol levels, blocked arteries, high blood pressure and heart disease. Saturated fat is mainly found in meat and dairy products. Unless you have a problem with cholesterol levels, it's not necessary for most people to totally eliminate saturated fat from their diet, as long as you are also eating a good range of EFAs and as long as fat doesn't make up too high a proportion of your total food intake. Total fat intake, including EFAs, should make up no more than 30 per cent of your diet and for anyone with a family history of heart disease, it should be much lower (less than 10 per cent).

But the biggest fat culprit, to be avoided totally, is:

Trans fatty acids or hydrogenated fat – these are the worst of all for health and ageing effects on your body. They begin as polyunsaturated vegetable oil but have hydrogen added to improve texture and increase shelf life. Small amounts of trans fats can be found in meat and dairy products, but the chemistry of naturally occurring trans fats is different from the man-made ones in processed foods and natural trans fats do not have the same negative effects on health.

Research suggests that trans fats:

- Are bad for your heart.
- Increase the risk of breast cancer.
- Block antioxidants from working in the body.
- Hinder the absorption of essential fatty acids.
- Some researchers believe they are almost impossible for the body to break down and so lead to weight gain which is hard to shift.
- There is so much concern over the effects of trans fatty acids on health in the US that from 1 January 2006 food companies have to label trans fat content on all foods.
- In Britain several companies have taken steps to reduce the amount of trans fats in products, but they are still present in many packaged foods and snacks.
- On food labels watch out for trans fatty acids, trans fats, hydrogenated fat, hydrogenated vegetable oil or hydrogenated oil – they are all different names for the same thing.
- As a general guide, caramel biscuits and chocolate bars often contain hydrogenated oils and can have a high trans fat content.
- Organic standards will not allow the inclusion of any trans fats.

Blood sugar levels

Sugar is one of the most ageing foods. It has a bad effect on energy levels and mood. It can also affect the digestive system, causing irritable bowel syndrome, bloating, stomach cramps and migraines. Sugar actively damages collagen production, which affects bones and tissues and causes skin to wrinkle and sag, all very obvious signs of ageing.

Many packaged foods contain high levels of hidden sugar but, in addition, refined, processed ingredients like flour are quickly broken down by the body into glucose, which is just another form of sugar. If you regularly feel sleepy and heavy after a meal it's probably because you've digested too much sugar from the food you've eaten.

The human body is designed to run on complex carbohydrates, proteins, fats and foods which release energy slowly:

⋯⋗ Lean meat, fish, eggs, nuts, whole grains, beans, lentils, vegetables and fruits are all good choices. These foods are converted into sugar more slowly by the body which means they provide a more consistent energy level and longer relief from hunger. This gives the body a better chance to actually use up food rather than turning it into fat.

⋯⋗ Say 'No' to simple carbohydrates and starchy staples. White bread, rice, pasta, potatoes and sugar all release their energy quickly, leading to substantial rises in blood sugar levels. The body often then over-compensates by releasing too much insulin which can lead to low blood sugar levels or hypoglycaemia. The swings in blood sugar levels, stimulating the over-production of insulin, stress the body and cause lethargy, fatigue and erratic moods. Ultimately, this can increase your chances of developing Type 2 diabetes.

DID YOU KNOW?
Eating too much sugar can trigger a process called glycation in the body. This results in stiffening tissues, and hardening joints and arteries. This is one of the main reasons for the serious health complications that are associated with diabetes.

The glycaemic index

Diet fads come and go but having a basic understanding of the glycaemic ranking of food seems to be useful. The glycaemic index ranks carbohydrates on the basis of their effect on blood sugar levels. Foods which are broken down quickly during digestion have a high glycaemic index and those which release sugar gradually and break down slowly have a low glycaemic index. The GI diet claims to be the least ageing way to lose weight or maintain a healthy weight because it establishes good eating habits with slow sustainable weight loss which doesn't stress the body or affect the metabolic rate. Its emphasis on fruits, veg, oats and whole grains makes sure the body is supplied with nutrients, including antioxidants and fibre.

Low GI facts:

- Low GI foods produce small rises and falls in blood sugar and insulin levels.
- Lower insulin levels are important for long-term health, as well as weight control, lessening the chances of diabetes.
- A diet rich in low GI foods can help gradual weight loss.
- Low GI foods will keep you feeling satisfied for longer. They can improve energy levels and combat lethargy.
- Fibre-rich whole grains, fruit and vegetables can help lower cholesterol levels.
- Balance is key. There are some high GI foods which provide essential nutrients. You should also always check the salt and fat content of packaged foods.

Some staple foods and their low GI alternative

High GI	Low GI alternative
Bread – white or wholemeal	Whole grain, stone ground flour, pitta bread, seed or fruit loaf
Cereal – processed sugary cereals	Porridge, oat-based cereals, muesli, bran
Potatoes – chips, jacket potatoes	Sweet potatoes, new boiled potatoes with skins, beans and pulses, whole grains like bulgar wheat
Rice – quick-cook varieties, sticky rice	Brown, whole grain or basmati rice, couscous, rice or udon noodles
Biscuits – most biscuits and cakes	Oat and dried fruit biscuits such as oatcakes, flapjacks and malt loaf

Mineral magic – chromium

┄┅► Studies suggest that chromium may enhance fat burning.

┄┅► Clinical evidence suggests that it reduces cravings and food binges, regulates blood sugar and evens out appetite.

┄┅► It's also thought to improve energy levels.

┄┅► Best results have been achieved with chromium picolinate but another form of the mineral, chromium polynicotinate, when bound with vitamin B3 also seems useful for reducing cravings and balancing blood sugar levels.

┄┅► Because it controls blood sugar levels, it is also part of the body's protection against diabetes.

┄┅► Chromium is difficult to absorb and only around 0.5 per cent of what's eaten is actually retained by the body.

┄┅► Boost your chromium intake by eating: beef, chicken, whole grain bread, oysters, eggs, peppers, nuts and beans.

DID YOU KNOW?
When you're hungry, tastebuds are more sensitive to sweet and salty tastes which is why many people choose unhealthy sugary or salty snacks. To combat these cravings, try eating six small meals a day to stop you feeling too ravenous.

DID YOU KNOW?
The UK government recommends eating five portions of fruit and vegetables a day to give you the vitamins, minerals and fibre you need for a healthy diet. The 5-a-day logo is now present on the packaging of foods which count towards your daily quota.

DID YOU KNOW?
Stress could be making you fat. When you're stressed, levels of the hormone cortisol rocket, causing blood sugar and insulin levels to rise. In turn this causes increased fat storage, high blood pressure and speeds ageing.

Vital vitamins and minerals

- The body's ability to digest food, breaking it down into sugar (or glucose) and releasing energy to body cells is dependent upon the presence of vitamins and minerals.
- Without them, less energy will be produced and there will be a greater tendency to lay down fat.
- The transport of glucose from the blood to the cells requires vitamins B3, B6, chromium and zinc.
- The further breakdown of glucose into energy requires vitamins B1, B2, B3, B5, and C, plus iron and co-enzyme Q10.
- Co-enzyme Q10 is a compound that is produced naturally in the body. It is used to promote cell growth, protect cells from damage and is important in the fight against ageing. The richest food sources are meat, poultry and fish, while other good sources include soya bean and canola oils, and nuts. There are also traces in fruit, vegetables, eggs and dairy products.
- Eating a range of fresh foods, including fruits and vegetables, proteins and fats will increase the variety of vitamins and minerals you consume.

Fibre, blood sugar and health

- Fibre is an essential part of a healthy diet and vital for your body to function properly.
- Fibre slows down the rate at which glucose is absorbed from food into the bloodstream. This gives the body more time to process carbohydrates, leading to lower blood sugar levels and better carbohydrate metabolism.
- One thing all good nutritionists agree on is that a high-fibre diet is one of the best ways to avoid putting on weight.
- Fibre keeps bowels regular and prevents your digestive system becoming sluggish.
- Wheat bran is one of the least effective forms of fibre and may prevent absorption of vitamins, minerals and other nutrients.
- The fibre present in oats, vegetables, fruit, lentils and other pulses is much more effective and kinder to your gut.
- Fibre is bulky and so helps you to feel full. The processed white versions of food are converted into sugar faster than their brown, less refined alternatives.
- Ensuring you eat an adequate amount of fibre will help to control blood sugar levels and avoid surges of sugar or insulin.
- Konjac fibre, derived from the Japanese konjac plant, absorbs ten times as much water as wheat bran and helps balance blood sugar levels. In Japan it's considered so effective it's used for the treatment of diabetes.

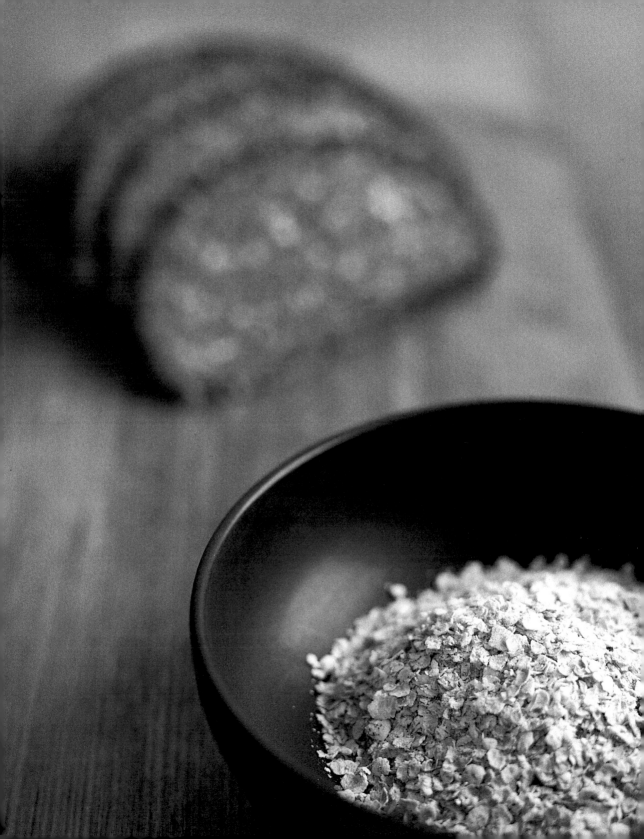

Variety is the spice of life

Nutritionists increasingly stress the importance of a varied diet. It is the best way to make sure you are eating all the nutrients your body needs to keep it working properly and in the right combinations. This ensures optimum absorption, which is vital if you want to slow the signs of ageing and the health problems associated with it.

A diet based around fresh food including fish, poultry, some lean meat, with plenty of fresh vegetables and fruit, whole grain cereals, and good fats will give you all the protein, fat, carbohydrates, fibre, vitamins and minerals your body needs.

It is becoming increasingly clear that simply adding supplements to your diet isn't enough. Nutrients need to be eaten in the right combinations if they are to be of any use, and eating them in fresh foods and varying your choices gives you the best chance of this.

FAT, PROTEIN AND CARBOHYDRATE – THE IDEAL COMBINATION
The average western diet derives 42 per cent of calories from fat, 15 per cent from protein and 43 per cent from refined carbohydrates. » Nutritionists calculate that the ideal diet should derive no more than 30 per cent of calories from fat, 15 per cent from protein and 55 per cent from complex carbohydrates.

DID YOU KNOW?
Researchers at Tufts University, Boston, Massachusetts claim the more variety there is in your diet, the more likely you are to lose weight.

Cut the calories and live longer?

Scientists are looking at the question of whether the simple secret to remaining youthful could be to eat less. We're not suggesting Kate Moss-thin limbs as research shows that crash dieting affects energy levels, brain function and mood and leads to older-looking skin. However, it is a fact that a typical Western diet supplies 40 per cent more calories than the body actually needs and overeating is one of the main causes of ageing and age-related illnesses. Studies suggest that a lower calorie diet may mean a longer, healthier life, perhaps because if you eat less the body produces more melatonin, a powerful antioxidant.

Dr Roy Walford, Professor of Pathology at the University of California, says that people may benefit by cutting their calorie intake by 10 per cent, but emphasizes that it's vital to choose food carefully to ensure an adequate supply of nutrients. He stresses the importance of eating a varied diet.

Researchers at University of Wisconsin-Madison Medical School in the US have also found that limiting calorie intake can slow normal age-related muscle loss. They have linked their findings with the fact that restricting calories may lower the production of harmful free radicals.

COMBINING WORKS WONDERS
A study at the University of Illinois in 2004 found that while the lycopene present in tomatoes provided protection against prostate cancer, if tomatoes were eaten with broccoli they offered even greater protection. » 'Separately, these two foods appear to have enormous cancer-fighting potential. Together, they bring out the best in each other and maximize the cancer-fighting effect,' says John Erdman, study leader, University of Illinois.

France vs America

In the diet stakes, France wins every time. The French eat a range of food, including butter, red meat, cheese and wine, and desserts and pâtisserie are not off the menu, at least at weekends. And yet the French remain slimmer than their American counterparts and suffer less from diet-related illnesses, including heart disease and diabetes. The key factor seems to be the quality of the food eaten – mainly fresh foods including fruit and vegetables with little reliance on convenience or fast food. French portions also tend to be smaller, but they take their time over meals and really enjoy what they eat.

The American diet, on the other hand, is generally very reliant on fast food and the super-size culture – the sort of meals that give an instant hit but leave you wanting more just an hour or so later.

Will Clower, a neuroscientist who wrote *The Fat Fallacy: The French Diet Secrets to Permanent Weight Loss* after living in France for two years, noted that when Americans went to live in France they tended to lose weight while the French who moved to the US usually put on weight.

DID YOU KNOW?
Researchers at the University of Pennsylvania and CNRS in Paris compared portions in fast-food outlets in Paris and Philadelphia and found the average American serving size was 25 per cent larger than the French.

DID YOU KNOW?
US Government surveys show that only 11 per cent of the French are obese compared with 30 per cent of Americans, and this is despite their well-known love of good food and wine.

Make the most of your meals

···> Take time over your meals and avoid rushing them.

···> Sit down but make sure you are upright and breathe properly
    to help digestion.

···> Ideally, only eat when you are relaxed and comfortable – this way
    you will be aware of what your body needs. You'll also enjoy your
    food more.

···> Chew each mouthful thoroughly and don't bolt your food – you'll
    find your meal much more satisfying. A good way to make sure you
    do this is to put down your knife and fork between mouthfuls – just
    remember those old etiquette books.

···> It may seem obvious, but stop eating when you begin to feel full.

···> Avoid grazing or boredom snacking. If you can't get by on three
    decent meals a day, try six smaller ones but always avoid snacking
    on rubbish. Healthy snacks like nuts, seeds and fruit will keep you
    satisfied, as well as supplying a range of anti-ageing vitamins,
    minerals and essential fats – they're good for your skin and bones,
    and even help you sleep.

'Food is one of the best pleasures
in life. We should not eat like
we're robots or on autopilot.'

MIREILLE GUILIANO, AUTHOR OF *FRENCH WOMEN DON'T GET FAT:
THE SECRET OF EATING FOR PLEASURE*

Food for healthy hair, nails and teeth

When assessing a patient's health, GPs and alternative practitioners will often look at the condition of their hair and nails. This is because they can both give a good indication of what's going on inside the body. A dentist will tell you the same. The state of someone's teeth and gums can give away a great deal about just how healthy or otherwise the person is. A key factor in this is good nutrition. It really is possible to eat your way to a younger-looking, healthier you.

Youthful hair

A young person's hair shines. It looks glossy and alive, it has movement. By contrast, we associate getting older with dull, brittle, static hair. That's even before you factor in the loss of colour, greying or problems of thinning hair. With a little know-how, you can tackle ageing hair problems from the inside before you turn to salon treatments.

Hair facts

···⟩ Hair is 97 per cent protein. The other 3 per cent is made up of amino acids, minerals and trace elements (including silica).
···⟩ The hair follicle is the base of the hair embedded in the scalp, where the cells form a bulb. The follicle is fed by a network of blood vessels.
···⟩ The hair is alive although there is no sensation or feeling.
···⟩ Hair is thickest when you are in your early 20s; after this the number of hairs on your scalp declines. At the age of 20, there are between 90,000 and 180,000 individual hairs, depending on hair colour.
···⟩ Average hair loss per day is between 100 and 125 hairs. Any more than this can lead to thinning.
···⟩ There is greater hair loss in spring and autumn as a natural response to changes in season and the amount of daylight – scientists have found people lose more hair in November than any other month of the year.
···⟩ Hair also grows more slowly in winter as circulation is generally more sluggish.
···⟩ Hair naturally thins as part of the ageing process. Just compare the figures: an average 20-year-old will have 600 hairs per square centimetre while the average 50-year-old will have less than half that figure.
···⟩ Hair loss is usually less of a problem for women as hair tends to thin evenly over the whole scalp rather than in distinct bald patches.

Youthful, healthy hair needs:
···⟩ Protein
···⟩ Iron
···⟩ Vitamins and minerals
···⟩ Essential fatty acids, especially Omega-3 and oleic acid (or Omega-9) which is most abundantly found in olive oil.

Avoid:
···⟩ Crash diets – they are a shock to the system and stress your body. They may well not meet your basic nutritional requirements, resulting in dull, lifeless hair, a loss of texture and sheen. You may even suffer temporary hair loss.

Ageing hair problems

Hair loss

While male pattern baldness is largely genetically programmed, temporary hair loss or thinning in women can have many causes and can be very upsetting.

There can be many reasons for hair loss, including hereditary factors, general health, emotional and physical stress, and taking certain drugs or medication. But nutrition can play an important part. In particular, crash diets, poor nutrition and extreme weight loss can result in thinning hair.

HAIR GROWTH
Stress can interfere with hair growth. There may be a three-month delay between the period of stress and hair loss, plus another three-month wait before significant regrowth. Stress does not cause permanent hair loss but it does affect the strength of the hair. » Hormones also affect hair growth, again in three-month cycles. This is especially noticeable during pregnancy and the menopause. » Thyroid misfunction can be another reason for problems, both when under- or overactive. » Certain commonly prescribed drugs can lead to temporary hair loss, including antibiotics, amphetamines and diet pills, antidepressants, beta-blockers, contraceptives, steroids, and vitamin A derivatives.

If hair loss is a problem:
- You may be anaemic – try adding iron-rich foods to your diet, in particular egg yolks, dark, leafy green vegetables and lean red meat.
- A zinc deficiency can also add to the problem, especially if your hair is very fine and breakable. Improvements may take several months to become obvious. To increase your zinc intake, see opposite.
- If you suspect that stress may be causing the problem, eat more vitamin-rich foods, concentrating on vitamins C and the B group as these will boost your immunity and support your nervous system.
- Try adding Royal jelly to your diet. Bee pollen is an amazing substance, packed with the nutrients we need for cell growth. It will help boost hair condition as it is an excellent source of pantothenic acid, which is also known as vitamin B5. This is particularly useful if you have been prescribed antibiotics, the contraceptive pill or sleeping pills.

DID YOU KNOW?
Peanut butter may help prevent baldness. Researchers have found that peanut butter contains a nutrient called inositol which has had some effect against male hair loss.

Greying hair

Grey facts:

- Roughly half the population has some grey hair by the age of 40.
- The rate of greying is mainly determined by genes.
- Some women find their first grey hairs in their teens, while others never go grey at all.
- A poor diet and stress can accelerate the rate of greying.
- Grey hair is not a reliable indicator of age but there's no doubt it is fundamentally linked with ageing.

Is your diet ageing your hair?

Alcohol can turn your hair grey. Drinking too much drains B vitamins from your body which can lead to premature greying.

Choose foods which are rich in B-complex vitamins to boost your hair colour:

- Liver and offal
- Brewer's yeast
- Raw wheatgerm
- Rice bran
- Brown rice
- Broccoli
- Spinach
- Eggs
- Royal jelly is also a good source of vitamin B5

Silica can also help slow the rate of greying. It is found in:

- Onions
- Oats
- Millet
- Barley
- Whole wheat
- Beetroot
- Horsetail herb

Zinc can also help maintain glossy hair colour. To bump up your zinc levels, eat:

- Oysters
- Crab
- Fish
- Meat
- Milk
- Egg yolks
- Mushrooms

DID YOU KNOW?
Liver is a particularly rich source of PABA (para amino benzoic acid) which is related to folic acid. It helps the body utilize protein and can delay signs of ageing, including correcting the loss of hair colour. PABA is also found in whole grains, raw wheatgerm and molasses.

Dry, lifeless hair

Gleaming, well-cut hair should be your crowning glory but environmental factors, the weather, central heating and diet can all take their toll and combine to drain the lustre from your hair, instantly ageing you no matter how good the rest of you looks.

To improve hair condition:

1 Drink plenty of water. Rehydrate your scalp and follicles and ensure the blood is circulating well to feed your hair with all those vital nutrients.

2 Increase your consumption of essential fatty acids. Snack on nuts and seeds and use good-quality olive oil for cooking. Dress your salads and vegetables with extra virgin olive oil and tasty nut oils.

3 Sulphur has been dubbed the beauty mineral, and among other uses it is important for glossy, smooth hair. It is found in vegetables like cabbage, broccoli, Brussels sprouts and horseradish root. You can tell if sulphur is present in vegetables by the smell when you cook them.

DID YOU KNOW?
When we are young, hair grows about 1cm (½in) per month, but as we age the rate of hair growth slows along with our metabolism and general rate of cell turnover.

DID YOU KNOW?
It's not just an illusion. Your hair really does grow faster in summer when weather is warmer and your circulation is less sluggish.

Dandruff

Dandruff occurs when the natural process of skin shedding on the scalp builds up into larger, more noticeable flakes. Despite appearing to be a dry skin problem, dandruff most often affects people with oily skin and hair. Scientists largely agree that it is caused by a tiny yeast-type fungus called Pityrosporum-ovale which is naturally present on everyone's scalp. Various factors can cause this fungus to multiply, leading to the inflammation and scaling associated with dandruff.

Seasonal weather changes can trigger flare-ups (the problem is usually worse in the winter), as can overactive oil glands, food allergies, stress and harsh hair products.

As well as using specific hair products, tackling the problem from the inside by adjusting your diet can make a big difference.

···⟩ Increase your intake of B vitamins – in particular wheatgerm, whole grains, cabbage, spinach, broccoli, eggs, fish, liver, chicken, lentils, beans and nuts.
···⟩ Cabbage, broccoli and eggs are especially helpful as they also include sulphur which is an excellent mineral for improving hair health. Onions and horseradish will also boost your intake.
···⟩ A deficiency of essential fatty acids has been linked to dandruff flare-ups. Include plenty of Omega-3 oils from fish, seeds and nuts.
···⟩ Garlic and the herb oregano have also been found to help.
···⟩ Remember that too much sugar, alcohol and stress can all deplete B vitamin levels.
···⟩ Food allergies can be a trigger and among the most common allergens for dandruff are chocolate, nuts and shellfish. It is worth keeping a food diary if you suspect anything you eat may be making the problem worse.

Healthy nails

Healthy-looking nails are important for creating a youthful impression. Bitten, broken, flaky nails just don't look good and can spoil your image. Obviously no matter how balanced your diet is, your nails won't look good if you bite them and don't give them a regular manicure. But eating the right things is a very good start.

Nail problems

Brittle, spoon-shaped nails can be caused by a lack of iron. The most easily absorbed form of iron is found in meat, offal, poultry, tuna and egg yolks. It is also present in small quantities in dark green leafy vegetables, grains, almonds, kidney beans and some fruits, including apricots. It's worth remembering that you will absorb more iron if a food source of vitamin C – for instance fruit or vegetables – is eaten at the same time.

White spots on the nails can be caused by bruising, but if you haven't knocked your nails recently, a zinc deficiency could be to blame.

When nails are cracked or flaking, try eating silica-rich foods. After all, silica is one of the main components of nails (see page 42).

To help nails grow smoothly and evenly, you need to increase the amount of sulphur-rich foods in your diet (good sources of sulphur include broccoli, cabbage, watercress, eggs, onions,meat, alfalfa).

For all round good condition and nail health, boost your intake of EFAs (see page 112).

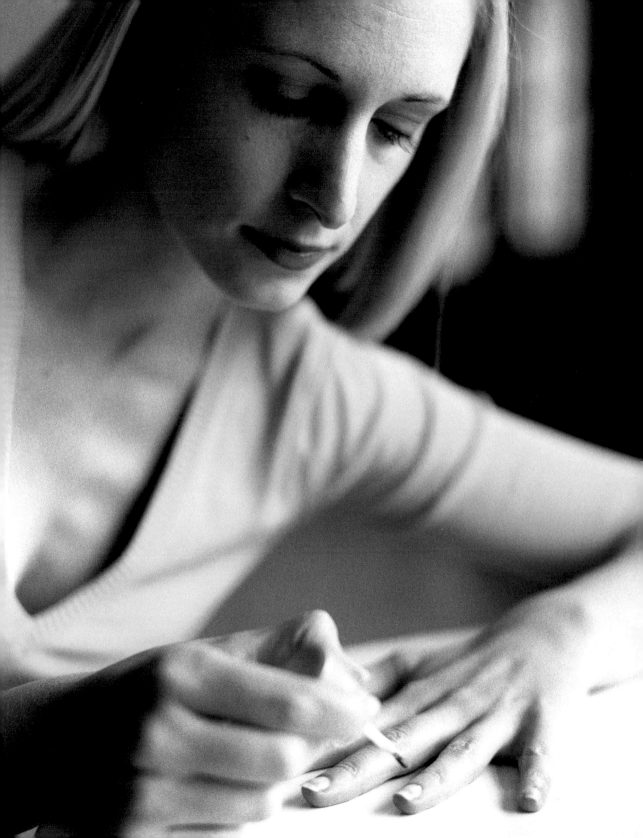

Healthy teeth

I'm not for one minute suggesting you aspire to a Hollywood-perfect smile, but as you age teeth begin to discolour and wear down. You may also notice other changes.

Ageing signs

⋯⋗ Teeth appear dull.
⋯⋗ They begin to develop halo shapes at the edge of the tooth which become very discoloured and make teeth look older.
⋯⋗ Gums shrink and lose their shape.
⋯⋗ Ageing, receding gums can give you a long-in-the-tooth look.
⋯⋗ Gums are prone to bleeding and puffiness, which can cause bad breath.
⋯⋗ Lips are also affected, especially if you are a smoker, as puckered lines appear around the mouth and at the corners.

Good oral hygiene and regular visits to the dentist are vital, I can't stress that enough. But your diet can really help you hold back the worst signs of dental ageing.

Calcium and vitamin D are vital for the development of strong healthy teeth and it is important to maintain a healthy, balanced diet to ensure you are receiving all the nutrients you need.

Good sources of vitamin D include:

⋯⋗ Sunshine
⋯⋗ Milk
⋯⋗ Eggs
⋯⋗ Sardines
⋯⋗ Tuna

The best calcium sources include:

⋯⋗ Milk and dairy products
⋯⋗ Yogurt
⋯⋗ Sardines and other fine-boned fish
⋯⋗ Tuna
⋯⋗ Almonds
⋯⋗ Spinach

Many of the most ageing dental problems are connected with gum disease. Making sure your diet includes plenty of foods rich in vitamin C will help you combat infection. Don't forget your body cannot store vitamin C. Any excess is lost in urine and so a fresh daily source is essential. Abundant supplies are found in most fruit and vegetables. Kiwi fruits, strawberries, citrus fruits and red peppers contain particularly high levels.

Boosting your immune system generally with B group vitamins is also helpful.

DID YOU KNOW?
If you can't clean your teeth after eating something sweet or acidic, finishing with a piece of hard cheese will help remove harmful debris and reduce damage.

Holding back the years

For teeth, delaying the effects of ageing is as much to do with what you avoid as what you actually eat.

For a whiter, winning smile

- Limit the amount of tea, coffee and red wine you drink and the dark-coloured foods you eat as these can all stain and discolour teeth making them look older.
- Do not smoke. It stains teeth, and causes periodontal wrinkles around the mouth which are extremely ageing. Smoking also depletes vitamin C and other nutrients, leaving you more at risk of gum disease and infections.

- Avoid fizzy drinks – the acid which creates the fizz attacks tooth enamel and encourages bacteria and decay.
- Cut out sugary drinks and foods. They also affect enamel and promote the growth of bacteria which causes gum disease and tooth loss.
- Remember that although fruit juice is healthier for your body the acid and fruit sugars it contains can still damage teeth.
- Chewy or boiled sweets are particularly bad for your teeth as they remain in your mouth for a long while. They are also often eaten over a long period of time rather than in one go which prolongs the time your teeth are under attack by raising damaging sugar and acid levels in your mouth for longer.

TAKE CARE OF YOUR GUMS
Dental health and hygiene are vital for the health of your heart too. The same bacteria that cause gum disease can trigger an immune response in the body leading to inflammation, including inflammation of the arteries. A recent study in Sweden confirmed the link between gum and cardiovascular disease.

'I always steer clear of sweets because I don't think there's any energy in them.' GWYNETH PALTROW

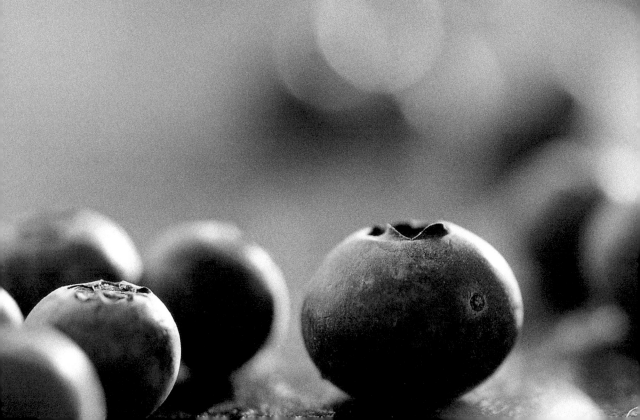

CHAPTER THREE

anti-ageing nutrients and super foods

There is... fix, no single miracle food that will turn
... the years and give you eternal youth, but there are
... amazing nutrients and foods that will do wonders
... importantly, your skin. If your skin is
... supple, glowing and radiant, then you'll
... younger. Sagging, dull, blotchy, wrinkly skin
... old and tired.

... there are foods that can accelerate the ageing process
by breaking down collagen and the infrastructure of
the skin, and foods full of fantastic vitamins, minerals,
antioxidants and essential fatty acids that can delay
the visible signs of ageing by destroying the destructive
agents we are exposed to every day. I call these foods
'super foods'. They are able to do what no amount of
cosmetic intervention can achieve; they help us preserve
what we've got so it looks good for longer. Make sure
your diet contains these every day and you're well
on the road to eternal youth.

The magic nutrients

It's the magic anti-ageing nutrients contained in the super foods that help keep you looking young. These are the key – the building blocks – to all super foods.

Antioxidants
⋯▹ Vitamin A
⋯▹ Vitamin C
⋯▹ Vitamin E
⋯▹ Carotenoids – beta carotene and lycopene
⋯▹ Flavonoids – resveratrol

Proteins
⋯▹ Essential amino acids
⋯▹ Nucleic acids

Essential fatty acids
⋯▹ Omega-3
⋯▹ Omega-6
⋯▹ Omega-9

Minerals
⋯▹ Selenium
⋯▹ Silica
⋯▹ Zinc

'It is good food and not fine words that keeps me alive.' MOLIÈRE

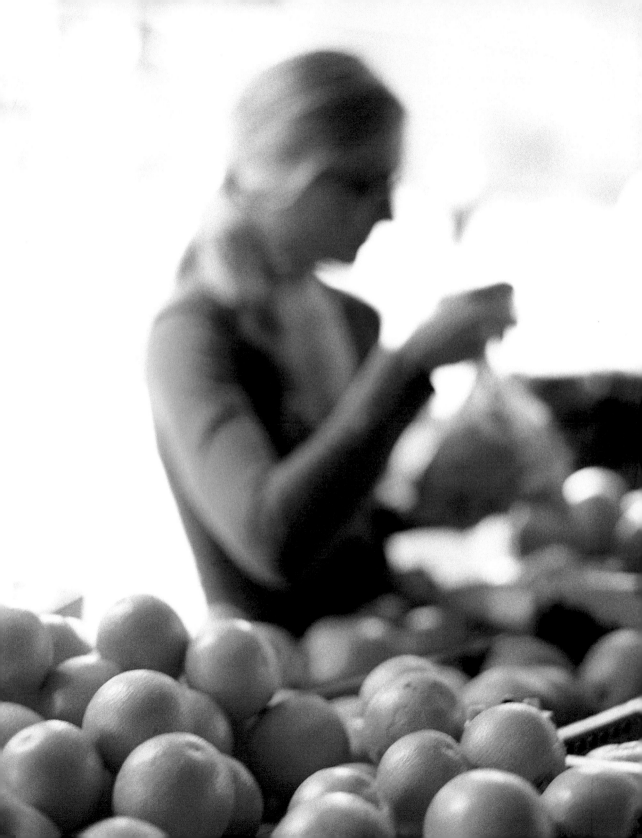

Antioxidants

⋯⋗ Antioxidants help repair the damage to our body cells. They are naturally occurring chemicals found in plant foods, such as fruit and vegetables.

⋯⋗ They are so called because they prevent a chemical reaction called oxidation. When we get stressed, our bodies produce free radicals and we're also being bombarded constantly by free radicals from polluted air, water and food. Oxidation is caused by these free radicals joining together and damaging our body cells and tissues.

⋯⋗ Free radicals accelerate ageing by destroying the collagen matrix in skin, thereby increasing susceptibility to developing wrinkles. Once our collagen-producing cells (fibroblasts) have been destroyed, they are gone for ever which is why it is so important to preserve what we have.

⋯⋗ Eating a combination of antioxidants is best because they all have different roles to play in preserving tissues and preventing disease. The most powerful anti-ageing antioxidants follow.

Vitamin A

⋯⋗ Comes in two forms: retinol ('animal' form found in meat, fish, eggs and dairy which the body can use straight away) and beta carotene (found in yellow, red, orange fruit and veg).

⋯⋗ Essential for reproduction and maintenance of epithelial tissue in skin.

⋯⋗ Keeps skin smooth and supple and known as 'the moisturizing nutrient'.

⋯⋗ Is fat soluble so can be stored in the body (mainly in the liver). Therefore some of the best sources also contain some fats and oils.

⋯⋗ Vitamin A combines well with vitamin E which helps protect and preserve vitamin A in the body.

⋯⋗ Not enough vitamin A means dry, wrinkly, rough skin.

⋯⋗ Good food sources: carrots, cabbage, kale, pumpkin, sweet potato, apricots, mango, spinach, peppers, eggs, liver (don't eat if pregnant), Parmesan cheese.

NB. Excess retinol can be toxic and dangerous for unborn children so pregnant women, or those trying for a baby, are advised not to follow a diet high in vitamin A.

Vitamin C

⋯⟩ Found in fresh fruit and vegetables.

⋯⟩ Needed for collagen and bone formation, and necessary for development and maintenance of connective tissue.

⋯⟩ Also has anti-inflammatory properties, speeds up production of new cells, keeps blood vessels healthy and boosts immune system – all of which keep skin looking great.

⋯⟩ Water-soluble so it can't be stored for long in the body and therefore needs replenishing daily.

⋯⟩ Easily destroyed by cooking and food processing.

⋯⟩ Best eaten with brightly coloured fruit and veg (the bioflavonoids responsible for the bright colours prevent vitamin C from being destroyed by oxidation).

⋯⟩ Eat with foods containing calcium (milk, cheese, yogurt, nuts, tofu, whole grains, etc) to enhance the absorption of vitamin C.

⋯⟩ Essential for drinkers and smokers whose bodies need more vitamin C than others.

⋯⟩ Not enough vitamin C means easily bruised skin, little red spots on the skin, fatigue.

⋯⟩ Good food sources: asparagus, broccoli, cabbage, blackberries, grapefruit, kiwi fruit, peppers, tomatoes, mango, melon, guava, oranges, pineapples, strawberries, limes, lemons, chillies.

Vitamin E

···⇢ One of the most effective antioxidants, attacking free radicals to prevent tissue and bone damage and the harmful effects of free radicals on the skin.

···⇢ Helps the body use oxygen properly.

···⇢ It maintains healthy muscles, nerves and reproductive systems, as well as protecting against ageing thread and varicose veins.

···⇢ Stored in the liver, in fat and muscle tissue but needs to be replenished regularly.

···⇢ Eat with vitamin C- and selenium-rich food to enhance absorption.

···⇢ Not enough vitamin E means varicose veins, thread veins, poor stamina, low libido.

···⇢ Good food sources: almonds, hazelnuts, peanuts, pistachios, sunflower seeds, soya beans, wheatgerm oil, prawns, avocados.

Beta carotene

···⇢ Beta carotene is the natural pigment (a carotenoid) found in bright yellow/orange and deep green fruit and vegetables.

···⇢ Carotenoids are able to protect against the damaging effect of sunlight.

···⇢ Once in the body, beta carotene is converted to retinol (vitamin A).

···⇢ Small amounts of fat are needed to convert beta carotene into the vitamin A the body can use (so, for example, sprinkle a dash of olive oil over a salad).

···⇢ It neutralizes free radicals and thus protects our skin's cell structure, slowing down the effects of ageing.

···⇢ Fantastic at boosting the immune system and protecting against damaging and ageing illnesses.

···⇢ Good food sources: carrots, apricots, sweet potatoes, kale, spinach, mango, cantaloupe melon, pumpkin, peaches.

Lycopene

⋯⋎ A red pigment (carotenoid) that occurs naturally in fruit and vegetables.

⋯⋎ Great for protecting the skin from degenerating, keeping the mind alert and the body functioning.

⋯⋎ Protects against the harmful rays of the sun.

⋯⋎ Powerful antioxidant so helps slow down and reverse the ageing of cells; great at deactivating ageing free radicals.

⋯⋎ Fat soluble so best absorbed when cooked with a little oil (or drizzled over a salad).

⋯⋎ Cooked tomatoes (eg tomato sauce, ketchup) have more lycopene per serving than uncooked.

⋯⋎ Good food sources: tomatoes (especially ripened on the vine), tomato paste, watermelons, pink grapefruit, guava, red peppers.

Resveratrol

⋯⋎ A natural chemical (flavonoid) found in fruits.

⋯⋎ Flavonoids protect the body against inflammation and boost the immune system.

⋯⋎ Resveratrol, in particular, appears to decrease the ageing of the DNA in the mitochondria, the energy plant of the cell.

⋯⋎ The darker the skin of the fruit, the more resveratrol it contains.

⋯⋎ Blueberries contain four times the amount found in other fruits.

⋯⋎ Good food sources: blueberries, cranberries, grape skins, red wine (in moderation!), peanuts.

DID YOU KNOW?
Salads sold ready chopped in bags have little or no flavonoid content.

Proteins

···❯ After water, protein is the next major component of our body. If we don't eat enough protein, our bodies will age more quickly. We need around 50,000 different proteins for our skin to create collagen, muscles, hormones, antibodies, enzymes and nerves. This is especially true for us as we age; over 30, it's important to have protein in your diet.

···❯ All proteins are built from a combination of 22 amino acids. Eight of these are 'essential' amino acids. To create protein, the amino acids link together to form chains (peptides). All eight essential acids must be present in the body in order for protein manufacture to take place so it's the *quality* of the protein we eat that is important and not the *quantity*. In charge of these complex protein-forming processes are nucleic acids – DNA and RNA.

···❯ The best-quality protein is from animal sources – fish, meat, game, eggs, dairy products; avoid eating too many red meats and full-fat dairy products because they contain saturated fat.

···❯ High-quality plant protein foods are soya, nuts, seeds, quinoa, wheatgerm, whole grains, brewer's yeast.

···❯ Lean protein (eg chicken breast, turkey breast, fish, eggs) is best.

···❯ The body can't store protein; the excess that isn't used to repair and rebuild the body is turned into fats and sugar.

···❯ Protein deficiency means rough skin, brittle nails, thinning hair, poor muscle tone, wrinkles and stretch marks.

'Protein is a rejuvenator.'
DR KURT DONSBACH, DONSBACH SCHOOL OF NUTRITION, USA

Essential amino acids

---» Maintain and repair cells throughout the body.

---» Eight amino acids are considered 'essential' because the body cannot manufacture them itself so we need to get them from food.

---» They are: isoleucine, valine, tryptophan, leucine, methionine, threonine, phenylalanine, lysine.

---» The body makes nucleic acids from the amino acids and nutrients in our diet.

> **DID YOU KNOW?**
> Protein-rich foods help make dopamine in the brain, which is essential for quick thinking, feeling alert and full of energy. They also release sugar slowly into the bloodstream so you don't get sudden blood sugar rushes. » Locusts are rich in protein … although I'm not suggesting you add them to your diet!

Nucleic acids

---» DNA (deoxyribonucleic acid) contains our genetic code and all the information needed for our bodies to grow, develop and function. DNA sends this information to the body via RNA.

---» RNA (ribonucleic acid) carries this information to the relevant cells.

---» Ageing is caused by cell degeneration. When DNA stops giving the orders to RNA, new cell construction stops and the ageing process accelerates.

---» By supplying the body with nucleic acids, you can look and feel 8–12 years younger than you actually are.

---» A diet rich in nucleic acids will give you more energy and your skin will look more youthful and healthier.

---» Good food sources of nucleic acids: wheatgerm, bran, spinach, asparagus, mushrooms, fish (especially salmon, sardines, anchovies), chicken liver, oatmeal, onions.

Essential fatty acids

Yes, fat is good for you. Well, the *right* kind of fat is good for you and can give you glowing, youthful skin and a great body. At least a third of our fat intake should be made up of polyunsaturated oils and another third by monounsaturated oils.

Our bodies can't manufacture EFAs so we need to get them from food. We need to eat a balance of the two to have the best anti-ageing effect on our skin; like an internal moisturizer, they keep skin looking wrinkle-free and healthy. The right balance is a ratio of 2:1 (two parts Omega-6 to one part Omega-3).

Stress is ageing and Omega-3 and 6 can lower the damaging chemicals that flood into our bloodstream when we get stressed. As we get older, levels of cortisol (one of the stress chemicals) rise in our body. This has the effect of making our cells resistant to insulin so our body fat increases. Keep eating omega rich foods to stay slim and svelte.

Omega-3

Important for healthy skin and bodies; Omega-3 is used to build cell walls, making them supple and flexible.

Powerful anti-inflammatory properties so great for combating the ageing effect on the skin.

Increases the body's metabolic rate to burn fat more efficiently.

Nowadays, our diets are low in Omega-3s, which are more prone to damage in cooking and processing than Omega-6.

The main Omega-3 fatty acid is alpha linolenic acid (ALA) which is converted by the body into eicosapentaenoic acid (EPA) and eventually into docosahexaenoic acid (DHA).

Good food sources: flax seed (oil and nuts), hemp seeds, fish (tuna, salmon, herring, mackerel, sardines), walnuts, brazil nuts, avocados, dark green leafy vegetables like kale and spinach.

Omega-6

⋯⋗ The main Omega-6 fatty acid is linoleic acid which is converted into gamma linolenic acid (GLA) and later synthesized with EPA from Omega-3 into eicosanoids.

⋯⋗ Great for skin (especially skin disorders like eczema and psoriasis) when combined with Omega-3.

⋯⋗ Good food sources: olives and olive oil, chicken, seeds, nuts, fruits, grains, raw sunflower seeds, evening primrose oil, borage oil, pumpkin.

⋯⋗ Avoid refined oils, such as sunflower, corn and soybean, as nutrient value may be lost.

Omega-9

⋯⋗ Contains oleic acid which helps Omega-3 penetrate cell membranes to deliver their positive anti-ageing effect.

⋯⋗ This is a monounsaturated fat.

⋯⋗ Technically this is not an EFA as, unlike Omega-3 and 6, our bodies can manufacture a certain amount of Omega-9 (as long as the two EFAs are present).

⋯⋗ Oleic acid keeps our cell membranes soft and moisturized, helping to reduce wrinkles and maintain a youthful complexion.

⋯⋗ Good food sources: extra virgin olive oil (contains 75 per cent oleic acid), olives, peanuts, avocados, cashews, pecans, macadamia nuts.

Minerals

⤑ Minerals are essential for pretty much every body process – from healthy skin, bones and teeth, to controlling blood sugar levels, boosting the immune system and carrying oxygen around the body. They regulate and balance our body chemistry.

⤑ Many people have low mineral levels in their diets because food is highly refined and processed and the minerals have been removed. We only need small amounts of certain minerals to keep looking young.

Selenium

⤑ Slows down the ageing process, boosts energy levels.

⤑ Great antioxidant; it helps remove free radicals from the body to protect against premature ageing.

⤑ Organic food has higher levels of selenium than other kinds.

⤑ Works best when combined with vitamin E.

⤑ A trace mineral so you only need a small amount daily.

⤑ Good food sources: sesame seeds, brazil nuts, wholemeal bread, sunflower seeds, canned tuna in oil, herring, kippers, mackerel, garlic.

Silica

--⟫ Silica has amazing anti-ageing properties.

--⟫ It increases the skin's elasticity, repairs brittle, cracked nails.

--⟫ Helps the skin to store moisture and so reduce wrinkles and skin problems; it can even reduce grey hair.

--⟫ Good food sources: barley, millet, oats, onions and whole wheat.

Zinc

--⟫ Another trace element.

--⟫ Essential for insulin production, taste, smell, natural resistance to infection.

--⟫ Boosts the immune system and, as part of the enzyme that metabolizes food, produces energy.

--⟫ Essential for the production of new collagen.

--⟫ Protects and repairs DNA.

--⟫ Zinc deficiency means brittle, cracked nails, damaged hair, slow healing of wounds, acne.

--⟫ Good food sources: oysters, sardines, crab, pumpkin seeds, eggs, liver, cheese.

'You only have to survive in England and all is forgiven you …if you can eat a boiled egg at ninety in England they think you deserve a Nobel Prize.'

ALAN BENNETT

The top 10 anti-ageing foods

I've always maintained that popping vitamin pills is never a substitute
for the real thing. So here are my top ten anti-ageing foods that are
guaranteed to make you look younger:

- Blueberries
- Water
- Prunes
- Salmon
- Broccoli
- Beans/lentils
- Pomegranates
- Avocado
- Green tea
- Yogurt

top of the list for antioxidant activity, these are *the* super food when it comes to slowing the ageing process. Blueberries have more antioxidants to protect every cell in the body than any other fruit or vegetable.

The dark pigments called anthocyanins are important antioxidant flavonoids which help protect and strengthen the walls of small blood vessels, preventing those nasty thread veins that appear as we get older. They also have a powerful anti-inflammatory effect. They're jam-packed full of vitamins C and E, fibre, potassium (good for our blood pressure), calcium and folic acid. Blueberries have extremely high levels of resveratrol (four times higher than cranberries).

They keep a young mind as well as a youthful body. A cup of blueberries a day is believed to improve short-term memory and protect against mental decline. They do wonders for your waistline; protect against heart and circulatory disease; protect against types of cancer; like cranberries, they can also help treat cystitis and other urinary infections. Sprinkle on breakfast cereals or whiz up in a blender with live yogurt for a tasty smoothie.

If you can't get blueberries, substitute the following:
- Cranberries
- Blackcurrants
- Blackberries
- Redcurrants
- Red grapes

DID YOU KNOW?
Blueberry jelly beans were created specifically for President Ronald Reagan.

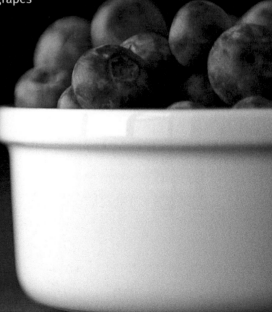

Water

···> This is a super drink rather than food –
it's easy to get hold of and it's free. Every
day, we lose around 10 cups of water from
our bodies. Drink at least 2 litres (4 pints)
of water, preferably still water, a day – that's
at least eight glasses.

···> Not too cold – because your body doesn't
waste energy having to heat it up you
absorb it much quicker.

···> Not flavoured water – that's full of sugar
and sweeteners.

···> Water is a vital nutrient. It makes up around
70 per cent of our body mass and is involved
in practically every body process.

···> All cellular hydration comes from the water
we drink, not from the moisturizer you put on
your face. Water literally hydrates the skin,
eliminating fine lines, flushing out harmful
toxins and reducing puffiness. Water boosts
our energy levels. It also swells the fibre we
eat which helps reduce bad cholesterol,
improves our digestion and enables us to
absorb nutrients more efficiently.

If you're dehydrated:

⋯⊁ Your skin will look older than it should.

⋯⊁ Blood is slower to carry vital oxygen and nutrients around the body.

⋯⊁ Your concentration levels are low and your metabolism is sluggish.

To check if you're dehydrated, pinch the back of your hand and if the skin sinks back slowly, you need a drink. Or just monitor the colour of your pee; the deeper it is in colour, the more dehydrated you are. A sign of good hydration is clear pee.

Don't wait until you feel thirsty because as you age your thirst mechanism fails to function as well as it should. I find that the more water I drink, the more thirsty I become, making it easier to keep on drinking. Drink water regularly for a week and you'll see an improvement in the mirror.

⋯⊁ Water, especially 'hard' water, contains important minerals, such as calcium and magnesium.

⋯⊁ It suppresses appetite naturally and helps our bodies use stored fat, helping you stay slim.

⋯⊁ Water maintains muscle tone because it allows muscles to do their job and contract naturally.

⋯⊁ Good sources of water (apart from bottled or tap): raw fruits and vegetables (carrots, watermelon, tomatoes, lettuce, apples, broccoli, grapefruit, cucumber).

DID YOU KNOW?
Water makes up between 50 and 60 per cent of your entire body weight. » A staggering 85 per cent of the brain is water and 75 per cent of the upper body's water is stored in the spine to cushion and protect it. » Every day you lose a cup of water through the soles of your feet and two to four cups simply through breathing. » Drinking a can of cola every day adds up to almost 32,000 calories a year – drink water instead and you'll lose 4kg without any effort.

'Water is the only drink for a wise man.' HENRY DAVID THOREAU

Prunes

⋯❯ The dried fruit of a plum tree, prunes have extremely high levels of antioxidants – eating just seven a day will give you all the antioxidants your body needs.

⋯❯ According to research from the US, prunes can protect against premature skin ageing thanks to the fact that they mop up more free radicals than any other fruit. And, yes, they do help to keep you regular.

⋯❯ More importantly, they have the highest ORAC score of any food – 5,770 units per 100g (see page 36) – which can help protect our bodies against cancers, heart disease and ageing.

⋯❯ Prunes are rich in potassium (good for high blood pressure), fibre, iron and vitamins A and B6. They are a good source of energy and easily digested.

If you can't get hold of prunes, try:
⋯❯ Dried apricots
⋯❯ Plums
⋯❯ Pears
⋯❯ Figs
⋯❯ Raisins

DID YOU KNOW?
Plum trees are grown in every continent except Antarctica.
» More than 70 per cent of the world's prunes are produced in California.

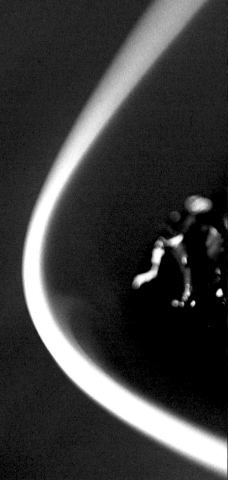

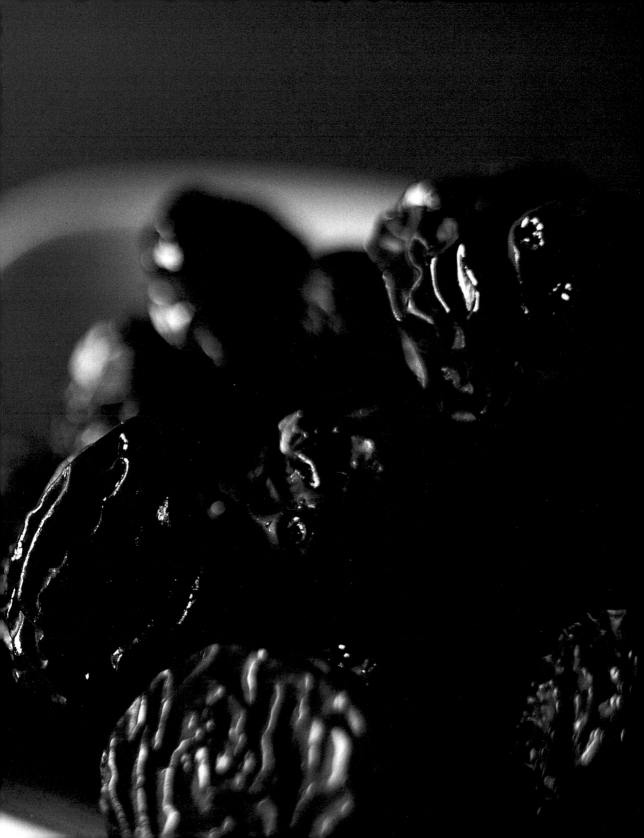

Salmon

···∤ Salmon meat contains DMAE (see pages 49 and 154), an antioxidant that stimulates nerve function and encourages the muscles under the skin to contract and tighten – better than a face lift? The DMAE stabilizes cell membranes and protects them from damage by free radicals.

···∤ Fish like salmon is an important source of essential Omega-3 fatty acids. If you're pregnant, the fatty acids are great for your baby's brain development. Omega-3 fats can also give you a mental boost, help you think more clearly and help you feel good about yourself. In addition to this, the Omega-3 is converted into prostaglandins which can combat dryness in the skin.

···∤ Like other oily fish, salmon contains copper (which helps produce melanin that protects our skin against the sun) and zinc which helps keep our collagen supply at maximum, reducing the effect of wrinkles and sun damage on our skin. It also improves the condition of our hair by strengthening the roots and encouraging natural oil production.

···∤ Salmon also contains protein. Healthy skin needs protein to keep producing healthy cells. It's also a great source of A, C and E vitamins and minerals (selenium, copper, zinc).

If you can't get hold of salmon, try:
···∤ Herrings
···∤ Anchovies
···∤ Mackerel
···∤ Trout
···∤ Sardines

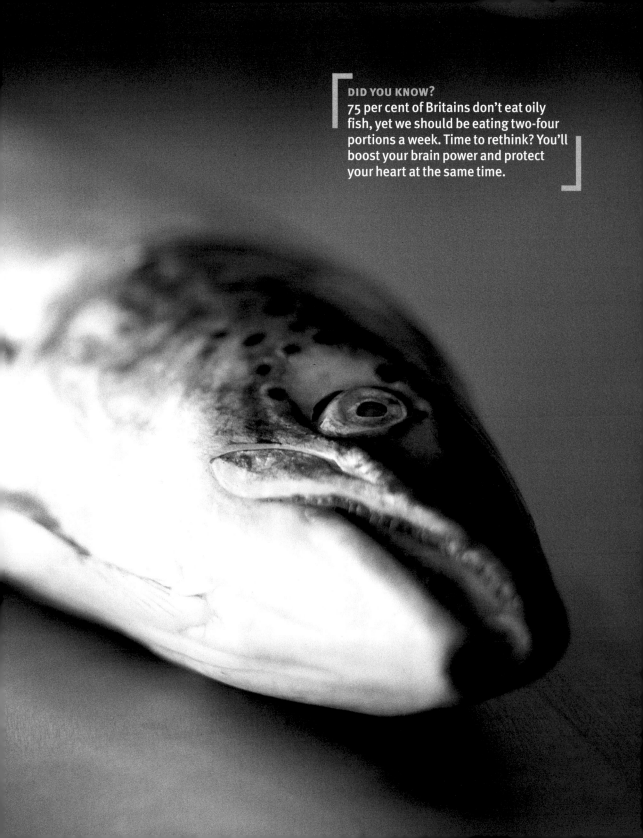

DID YOU KNOW?
75 per cent of Britains don't eat oily fish, yet we should be eating two-four portions a week. Time to rethink? You'll boost your brain power and protect your heart at the same time.

Broccoli

A cruciferous vegetable like kale, cabbage and Brussels sprouts, broccoli contains a great antioxidant called sulphoraphane. This antioxidant detoxifies and eliminates harmful free radicals. If you combine it with selenium (found in oily fish, tuna, game, brazil nuts, sunflower seeds, onions and garlic) it's 13 times more effective at fighting the free radicals that cause ageing.

It has an unusually high protein content which is good for maintaining healthy cells. There's a useful amount of fibre in this veg too. It's a great way to stimulate and detoxify the digestive system and the liver. If you can keep the toxin levels down in your body, your skin benefits too, looking clear and healthy.

Don't just eat the florets; use the leaves because they contain more carotenoids (protective chemicals that boost the immune system and fight ageing illness and infection) than the florets. Steaming is the most effective way of cooking broccoli because you retain all the great nutrients.

Rich in vitamin C (contains more vitamin C than oranges).

Full of beta carotene which the body converts into vitamin A – helps keep the skin looking good, especially if you've got acne.

Full of iron and chlorophyll to purify the blood.

Contains folic acid which aids the production of serotonin, a mood-enhancing chemical which makes us feel good in ourselves.

If you can't get hold of broccoli, try:

- Brussels sprouts
- Spinach
- Cabbage
- Kale
- Cauliflower
- Spring greens
- Asparagus

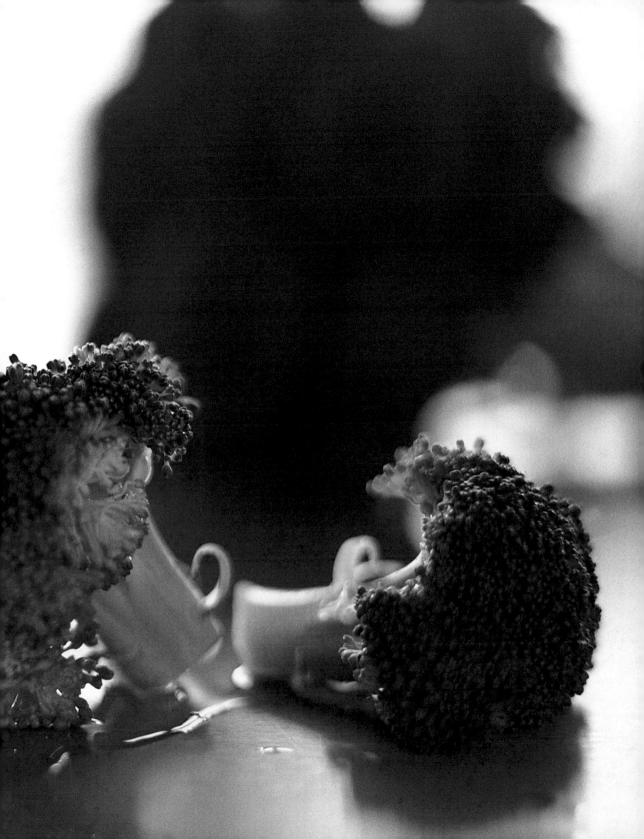

Beans and pulses

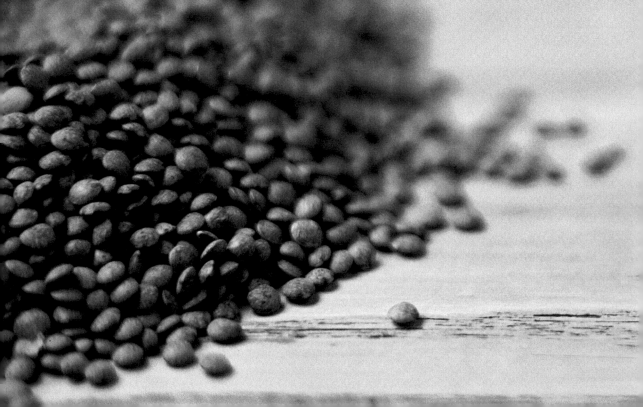

⇢ Eating beans and pulses stimulates the production of hyaluronic acid (HA). HA retains water in the skin cells so it acts as a moisturizer, keeping skin smooth and wrinkle-free. As we age, HA starts to decrease so we need to replenish it regularly.

⇢ Our bodies digest beans slowly which means a gradual increase in our blood sugar levels, rather than dramatic highs and lows. This means that we need less insulin to control the blood sugar. Too much insulin can have an ageing effect on our skin.

⇢ Beans and pulses are also a great source of fibre. Studies have found that eating at least 25g of fibre a day gives you a real age up to three years younger than someone who only eats 12g a day – which is the national average. You find fibre in plant foods; it contains no calories but makes you feel fuller sooner – which helps control overeating.

⇢ Pulses are members of the legume family (such as peas and green beans). If you combine them with wholegrain cereals you add the missing amino acids and so give a more balanced meal.

⇢ If you soak beans in water they become more easily digestible (and reduce their rather 'windy' properties). Soak them and then change the water before cooking them.

⇢ Beans have high levels of boron which is a great brain-booster, keeping us alert and our memory sharp.

⇢ Bean sprouts have high levels of vitamin C.

⇢ Pulses contain high levels of protein which we need for healthy collagen production and new cells to keep our skin looking well moisturized.

⇢ Soya beans, the best vegetable source of proteins, are also full of powerful antioxidants which prevent free radical damage.

Choose from:

⇢ Chickpeas	⇢ Butter beans
⇢ Kidney beans	⇢ Broad beans
⇢ Lentils	Peas
⇢ Soya beans	Baked beans
⇢ Mung beans	

DID YOU KNOW?
Collagen literally holds your skin together and is found in skin, tendons and bones. » Vitamin C is essential for its production. » Hyaluronic acid moisturizes the skin from the deeper layers to the outer. » Zinc increases hyaluronic acid and collagen levels in the skin.

DID YOU KNOW?
To remove the seeds from a pomegranate,
leaving the pith behind, cut it in half. Hold one
half, cut side down, over a bowl and then rap it
firmly with a wooden spoon a few times until
the bright seeds begin to rain down.

Pomegranates

···> Traditionally, the Ancient Greeks used
them to treat tapeworms. Now, they are
a big favourite of celebrities who have
known about the anti-ageing properties
of pomegranate for some time.

···> Pomegranate juice has more antioxidants
in it than either red wine or green tea. It also
contains high levels of ellagic acid, another
antioxidant, which boosts the skin's natural
defences against the sun. And we all know
how damaging – and ageing – the sun can
be. This is a natural stress reliever – great
for our hectic lifestyles and neutralizing
damaging free radicals.

···> As well being packed full of vitamin C and
potassium, pomegranates are a good
source of fibre so they help the digestion
and eliminate toxins.

···> You can now find pomegranate juice in most
major supermarkets.

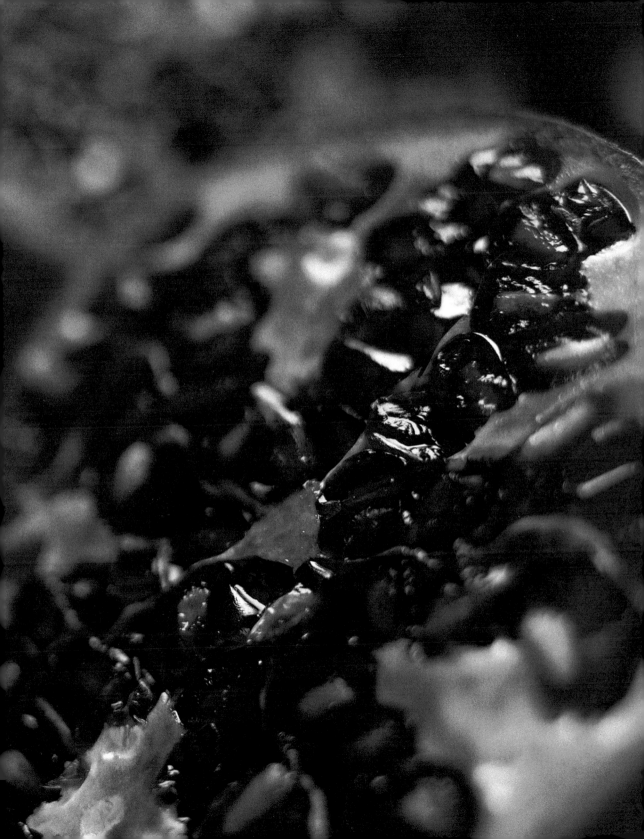

Avocados

⋯ Avocados have suffered in the past from a 'fat' image. People avoid them because they believe the fat is bad for them and they'll put on too much weight. Yes, avocados are quite high in fat but it's the 'good', monounsaturated kind which contains no cholesterol. More importantly, avocados are a brilliant source of vitamin E – a great antioxidant and the ironer out of wrinkles.

⋯ Like olive oil, they contain the handy Omega-9 essential fatty acid – oleic acid. Once again, a great antioxidant and protector against disease, cancer and strokes. They also contain some Omega-3.

⋯ They are a good source of potassium which helps the body eliminate waste and toxins, gives an oxygen boost to the brain (so great for keeping our minds sharp) and helps digestion by stimulating the stomach secretions.

⋯ If you eat an avocado with another vegetable or salad you will take in four times more lutein, eight times more alpha-carotene and 13 times more beta carotene which are all brilliant for eyes. It's also full of vitamin B6 and a good source of chromium (low chromium levels mean your hunger pangs are stimulated more) and helps to reduce PMS (eat regularly 10 days before your period).

⋯ Avocados also contain mannoheptulose, a special kind of sugar which, unlike ordinary sugar, doesn't stimulate insulin production.

⋯ Avocados are good for us both inside and out. They contain folate which is essential for cell regeneration. Eat them or mash them up with a dollop of live yogurt as a face mask. The extra collagen will reduce your wrinkles and give your skin a youthful glow. If you don't fancy the face mask, make a bowl of guacamole instead.

⋯ They are also a good source of fibre and antioxidant vitamins A, B6 and E.

⋯ Vitamins A and E can help reduce wrinkles.

⋯ Avocados contain an amino acid called tryptophan which is used by the body to make the mood-boosting chemical serotonin.

They are a good source of protein and easily digested.

If you can't get hold of avocados, try:
⋯ Kiwi fruit
⋯ Pumpkin seeds (for vitamin E)
⋯ Tomatoes (for potassium)

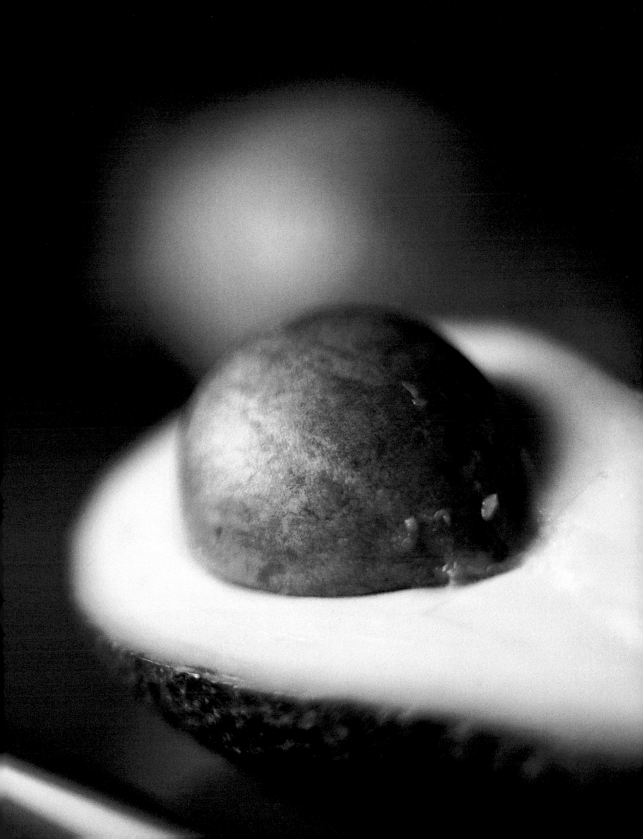

Green tea comes from the same plant as the more familiar black tea. The difference is that the leaves are steamed or pan-fried rather than fermented (as with black tea). It has lower levels of caffeine than black tea and higher levels of powerful antioxidants (polyphenols and flavonoids).

···> Flavonoids are used by plants to protect themselves against the damaging effects of UV light. Since green tea is rich in flavonoids, it can help protect the skin against ageing as well as reduce skin damage caused by the sun.

···> Green tea is one of the richest sources of antioxidants (30 per cent of the weight of a green tea leaf is made up of antioxidants). Research found that women with ovarian cancer who drank at least one cup of green tea a day had 44 per cent more chance of surviving cancer than women who didn't drink green tea. And if something's powerful enough to fight cancer, it's more than a match for keeping the skin looking good.

It has been shown to boost the metabolism, increase energy production and breaks down the fat stored in the body. It's also an anti-inflammatory – either as a drink or applied onto the skin directly.

···> Studies also show that green tea can strengthen bones and reduce the risk of fractures – ideal as we get older. It can also reduce gum disease and it contains fluoride to reduce tooth decay. It's even got a natural antihistamine which can prevent hayfever attacks.

···> Don't add milk to your tea; it cuts down the effectiveness of the antioxidants.

···> Tea also contains vitamin E – important for healthy skin.

···> Speeds up the metabolism so you burn off more energy.

···> If you use tea bags, remember to squeeze the bags to release all the antioxidants.

While I'm on the subject of tea, Rooibos tea is a traditional South African drink so I'm bound to be a fan. It's been shown to protect against the changes in cells caused by pollutants such as cigarette smoke and sunlight which are damaging to our skin. It's low in tannin and caffeine free. It can calm an upset stomach, skin rash or colicky baby. Put it on the shopping list.

If you can't get hold of a cup of green tea, try:
- Herbal teas, such as peppermint, chamomile, ginger
- Rooibos tea
- Or make your own – try warm water with a squeeze of lemon juice or grated ginger

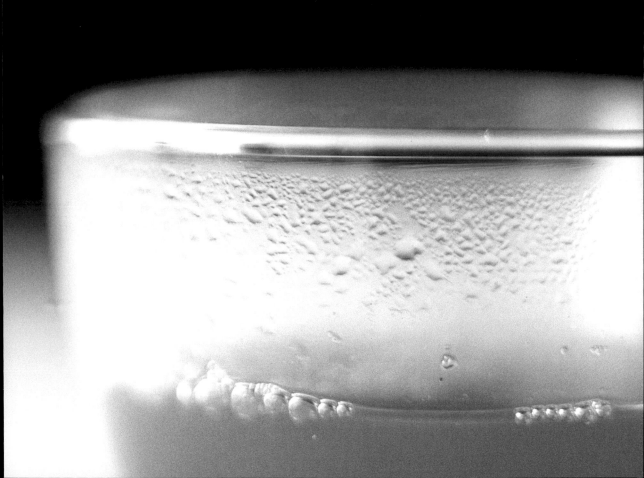

Live yogurt

⋯⋗ Yogurt started life as milk. Special probiotic cultures are added to heated milk and then allowed to incubate. These bacteria – including Lactobacillus bulgaricus, Lactobacillus acidophilus and Streptococcus thermophilus – aid digestion by helping the gut to do its work. And if your digestion is working properly, you'll be able to process all these great super foods efficiently.

⋯⋗ Yogurt contains protein, so will help provide the essential amino acids that the body needs. Easily digested (around 91 per cent compared with only 32 per cent of regular milk), live yogurt is a good substitute for people who are lactose-intolerant because it produces an enzyme called lactase, which breaks down lactose (which is the sugar in the milk).

⋯⋗ A daily dose of live yogurt can also banish bad breath. A study found that people who ate or drank around 75ml (3fl oz) of yogurt twice a day had significantly less hydrogen sulfide in their mouth which is a big cause of bad breath. Levels of plaque and gingivitis were also notably reduced in the mouth of the yogurt-eaters.

So what has bad breath got to do with feeling and looking younger? Gingivitis and periodontal disease causes ageing of the immune and arterial systems. It's believed that toxic bacteria can travel into the bloodstream, causing inflammation throughout the body, including the arteries. Only 21 per cent of us floss regularly. Regular brushing and flossing could knock six years off your biological age.

And while I'm on the subject of cleaning your teeth, don't brush your teeth straight after a meal. According to the British Dental Association this can do more harm than good, particularly after eating or drinking acidic foods, such as citrus fruits or fruit juice. These soften the tooth enamel so brushing too soon afterwards could attack it even more. Instead wait at least 20 minutes before you brush or nibble a small piece of cheese.

If you can't get hold of yogurt, try:
⋯⋗ Buttermilk
⋯⋗ Cheese (sheep's or goats')
⋯⋗ Low-fat cottage cheese

DID YOU KNOW?
Four out of five adults in the UK have gum disease (British Dental Association).

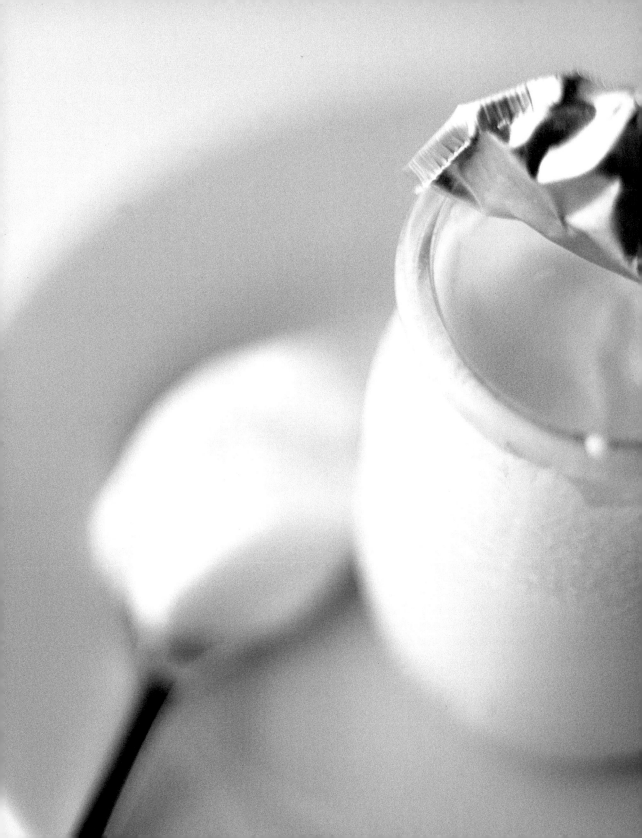

Fab foods

The following foods didn't quite make it into the top ten but should still be part of your weekly diet. They also contain powerful concentrations of our super nutrients:

---> Grains
---> Nuts and seeds
---> Oils
---> Fruit
---> Vegetables
---> Herbs and spices

Grains

Oats

···⇢ A bowl of porridge in the morning is a great way to start the day. Oats have a low glycaemic index (see page 84) so you get a slow release of sugar into the blood. This means a sustained insulin response which is much better for your skin as insulin destroys collagen, resulting in wrinkles and loss of elasticity.

···⇢ Add a dollop of Greek yogurt to your breakfast bowl and the fat and protein combine to slow down the absorption of carbohydrates even more. High-fibre foods, particularly soluble fibre like oats, help to keep your weight steady, reduce cholesterol and aid digestion. They reduce sugar, caffeine and nicotine cravings (all ageing). Oh, and they're good for your concentration, can help reduce the effects of a hangover and, thanks to the high levels of vitamin B6, do wonders for your sex life. Need I say any more?

Barley

It won't necessarily be in everyone's store cupboard, but barley is an easy way to get a great energy boost and, thanks to the silica it contains, does wonders for your skin, hair and nails. Choose from pearl barley, where the hull and bran have been removed, or preferably whole pot barley. Pearl barley has had around 60 per cent of its vitamin B removed – a bit like using white flour, rather than wholemeal.

Millet

Like barley, not something everybody has in their kitchen but worth adding to your shopping list. Millet contains silica which we need to make collagen for healthy skin, hair and nails. It's easy to digest and doesn't cause bloating. Because it isn't highly refined, like some flours, millet keeps all the essential nutrients. You can add millet to soups or casseroles; millet flour can be used in baking.

'A grain, which in England is generally given to horses, but in Scotland supports the people.'

SAMUEL JOHNSON

Nuts and seeds

Almonds

Hands up who's got almond oil in their bathroom cabinet? Yep, it's great for the skin and can help prevent stretch marks and scarring but it's good for our insides as well. Almonds are full of vitamin E which is great for holding back the years. They also have the most calcium of all nuts (good for bones) and a third more protein (good for maintaining skin cell structure) than eggs. Take a tip from ayurvedic medicine: to give yourself an energy boost in the morning, soak six almonds in water overnight and then eat them first thing for a powerful shot of protein, iron, calcium and potassium.

Walnuts

Full of the feel-good, mood-enhancing neurotransmitter serotonin, walnuts are also an important source of Omega-3 fatty acids, vitamin E and zinc – so great for healthy skin. Eat a handful of walnuts (about six) before a meal so you are getting a small portion of unsaturated fat; this slows down the emptying of the stomach so you'll feel full on less food. Eating sensible amounts of food means you won't pile on the pounds and you'll keep a more youthful figure.

Brazil nuts

These contain the highest natural source of selenium which can destroy free radicals caused by pollution, such as cigarette smoke. Whether you indulge in cigarettes or not (and I hope you don't!), the smoke is incredibly drying and ageing. Selenium is also responsible for manufacturing a powerful antioxidant that protects skin from damaging ultraviolet light. Brazil nuts are also a superb source of vitamin E which is great for the skin. Just a small handful a day will do the trick. They are a good source of protein and are great at giving an energy boost when we need it. Brazil nuts also contain vitamin C which helps our immune system.

Oils

Olive oil

Moisturizers are full of ingredients that mimic the body's attempts to prevent skin from drying out. But there are natural ingredients, like olive oil, that do exactly the same job. Full of vitamin E and Omega-9, olive oil is fantastic for your skin. It strengthens the collagen in skin to keep it looking young and healthy. In addition, a high level of olive oil in your diet, combined with fruit, vegetables, fish, nuts and whole grains, will cut the risk of premature death by up to 25 per cent – and I don't know anything more anti-ageing than reducing the risk of premature death! Choose extra-virgin olive oil – it's packed with antioxidants.

Flax seed oil

A powerful source of Omega-3 and 6 – essential fatty acids which are vital for healthy skin, hair and nails. Omega-3 also helps burn off carbohydrate calories quickly. It is a good source of magnesium which will help clear your head and lift a bad mood. Looking grumpy is *so* ageing! Use as an oil in dressings or sprinkle the seeds over salads, soups or your breakfast cereal.

'Life expectancy would grow by leaps and bounds if green vegetables smelled as good as bacon.' DOUG LARSON

Fruit

Apples

Apples are a great source of powerful anti-ageing antioxidants (called flavanols). They are great detoxifiers so give your skin a healthy glow. A recent American study found that people who replaced sugary sweets in their diet with apples lost an average of 6.75kg (15lb) in 12 weeks. Keeping your youthful figure will knock the years off you. Apples are also packed with fibre (pectin) which aids digestion and helps lower cholesterol. And they're great at banishing cellulite and detoxifying the body. And let's face it, this is one of the easiest foods to eat – no preparation, no fiddly cooking. Just wash and go.

Lemons

Full of B vitamins, carotene and vitamin C, as well as very high levels of polyphenols which are among the most powerful antioxidants. Great for fighting damaging free radicals which can speed up the ageing process. Begin the day with a glass of warm water and lemon juice to kick-start your digestion. The lemon juice helps to increase the skin's natural elasticity while the warm lemon water will go straight through your body, helping to purge all those ageing toxins.

DID YOU KNOW?
The Romans believed lemons were an antidote to all poisons. » Oranges don't ripen after they're picked but lemons do.

DID YOU KNOW?
An apple a day keeps the doctor away. It seems that eating apples really does help you stay healthy. Researchers have found people who eat more apples have fewer colds and respiratory problems. Pectin, the fibre contained in apples, aids digestion as well as lowering cholesterol. Studies in the US showed people eating three apples a day actually lost weight.

'Comfort me with apples:
for I am sick of love.'

THE SONG OF SOLOMON 2:5

Mango

They're a better source of beta carotenes than apricots or cantaloupe melons. The darker the colour of the fruit, the more beta carotene it contains. Half a mango will make up one of your five-a-day portions of fruit and veg. Full of vitamins A, C and E, they will mop up damaging free radicals to keep the body's tissues healthy and intact. Mangoes are good at helping to digest fatty foods. Their detoxifying properties have a positive effect on skin, improving the texture, reducing wrinkles and giving a youthful glow.

Guava

With five times as much vitamin C as an orange, guavas pack a hefty antioxidant punch. Even after canning, where they lose 25 per cent of the vitamin, guavas are a great source. Vitamin C is vital for the production of collagen and healthy skin and tissues.

Papaya

A powerhouse of beta carotene and vitamin C, so good for the immune system and great-looking skin. You'll find it is being used more and more in skin cream. Papayas contain an enzyme called papain which helps digest proteins needed for the healthy production of collagen. Try to eat fresh papayas because the antioxidants are pretty much lost in the canning process.

Strawberries

Strawberries contain something called ellagic acid which has been found to minimize the damage caused by pollution and smoke. They are great for cleansing our whole system, combating high blood pressure and keeping our skins looking glowing and healthy. They've long been believed to reduce wrinkles and benefit the complexion. They have more vitamin C than any other berry, which keeps the tiny blood vessels strong, preventing unsightly bruising and thread veins.

DID YOU KNOW?
The 'Paisley' design motif is a design from India based on the mango.
» More fresh mangos are eaten every day than any other fruit in the world.

Tomatoes

Yes, technically tomatoes are a fruit rather than a vegetable. They contain all the important antioxidant vitamins A, C and E. Tomato juice is a rich source of beta carotene which can slow down – and may even reverse – much of the ageing process. Lycopene is the antioxidant that gives tomatoes their red colour. Studies show that the higher the level of lycopene in your blood, the lower your risk of heart disease and stroke. Strangely, this is one food that improves its health benefits with cooking; cooked or processed tomatoes have more lycopene than fresh. And big isn't always the best. A study from the University of Glasgow found that cherry tomatoes had higher levels of antioxidants than other varieties.

⋯⋙ Eat with spinach, which is full of vitamin E, to reduce bad cholesterol.

⋯⋙ Avoid tomatoes if you're trying to give up smoking; they're related to the tobacco plant so might just stimulate your body's need for nicotine. Cut out tomatoes until your cravings have passed – about eight days after your last cigarette should do it.

DID YOU KNOW?
There are at least 10,000 varieties of tomato.

'A world devoid of tomato soup, tomato sauce, tomato ketchup and tomato paste is hard to visualize.'

ELIZABETH DAVID, *AN OMELETTE AND A GLASS OF WINE*

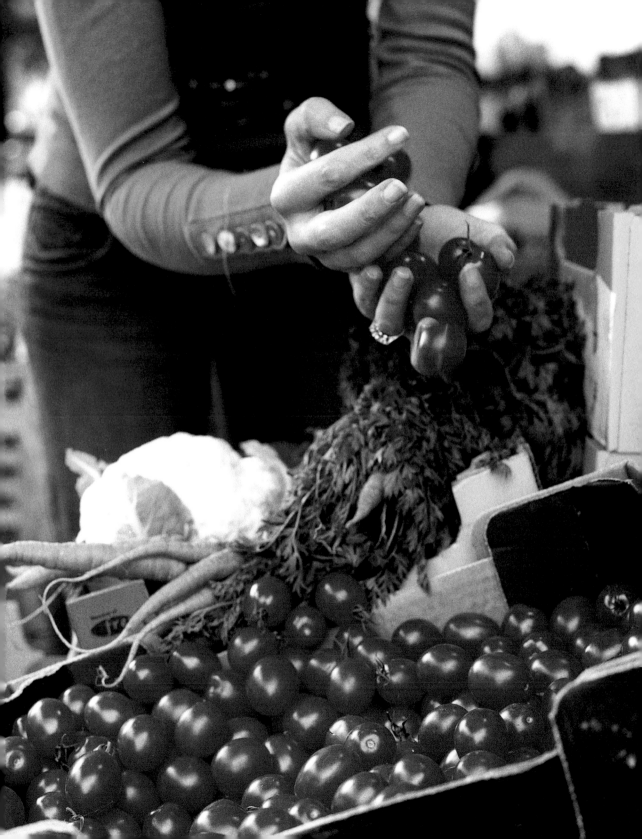

Vegetables

Beetroot

Has a high antioxidant content and is great at cleansing our bodies. Good source of beta carotene and vitamin C. The red colouring contains flavonoid anti-carcinogens which are also responsible for increasing the cellular uptake of oxygen by around 400 per cent. The more oxygen our cells get, the better they are able to detoxify themselves, the healthier we are and the younger we look. The more oxygen we get to our cells, the more colour we have in our skin and we all know rosy cheeks mean youthful looks. Beetroots contain iron and natural sugar which are great energizers and help improve the memory. Beetroot juice, if you can stomach it, is a good way to kick-start the system in the morning.

Carrots

Full of beta carotene which boosts immunity and neutralizes the damaging effect of free-radicals. Carrots are great at detoxifying the body. Research shows that eating carrots increases red blood cell levels and protects our skin against the damaging effects of the sun. So eat carrots to stay wrinkle-free. Carrots also contain vitamin A which (yes, your granny was right) can help you see in the dark; one carrot will give you all the vitamin A you need for a single day. Juice a couple of carrots with an apple for a great skin tonic.

⟶ The darker orange the carrot, the more beta carotene it contains.

⟶ You get higher levels of vitamin C in uncooked carrots, but more beta carotene in cooked carrots.

'I never worry about diets. The only carrots that interest me are the number you get in a diamond.' MAE WEST

Spinach

Like all dark green vegetables, spinach is full of wonderful micronutrients. Well known for being an excellent source of iron (so good for vegetarians) and folic acid (great for pregnant women), spinach also contains many protective carotenoids, such as lutein and zeaxanthin which are good for healthy eyesight. Use them in salads. Baby spinach leaves have 90 per cent more antioxidants than an iceberg lettuce. Also, combined with lycopene (found in tomatoes), it's been found to halve 'bad' cholesterol and reduce the risk of heart disease.

Cabbage

Forget soggy cabbage and school dinners. This powerful vegetable is worth putting back on the menu. All forms of cabbage contain compounds which help stimulate enzymes in your stomach and liver which filter out toxins that damage your health and speed up the ageing process. In Chinese cooking, pak-choi is well known for its detoxing properties. Try sauerkraut if you really were traumatized by school dinners. You can also place a cabbage leaf in your bra if you get mastitis when breastfeeding! Cabbage is full of vitamins A and C, beta carotene, folic acid and fibre.

Peppers

Peppers are a good source of antioxidants but the red ones are the superstars of the family. High in vitamins A, C and E as well as carotenes, peppers reduce the risk of developing cancer, heart disease, stroke and cataracts. In fact, peppers will give you twice as much vitamin C as an orange. Vitamin C is essential for giving us energy and boosting the immune system. Eat them raw in salads for the best effect.

⋯⇢ Peppers keep their vitamin C for weeks, especially if you store them in the fridge.
⋯⇢ Full of antioxidants which protect against cancer, arthritis and heart disease.
⋯⇢ Contain iron and potassium.

Sweet potatoes

Orange skinned sweet potatoes are rich in the anti-ageing, antioxidant beta carotene, as well as vitamins A, B, C and E. The beta carotene is stored in the fat layer of our skin and protects against the damage from the sun's ultraviolet rays.

DID YOU KNOW?
Recent studies suggest eating lots of cabbage is the reason for the low rate of breast cancer among Polish women.

Herbs and spices

Spices are an excellent way to liven up the taste of foods and make them more interesting. Varying flavours keeps tastebuds stimulated and means you're more likely to feel satisfied after eating. But a growing number of studies suggest that spices are about a lot more than just flavour and can play an important role in keeping you young and healthy.

DID YOU KNOW?
The active properties found in many spices decline when they are ground. To preserve their potency, grind your own as you need them.

DID YOU KNOW?
Curcumin can suppress blood vessel growth to tumours, effectively starving them.

Turmeric

There has recently been a great deal of excitement about curcumin, which is found in turmeric, the spice that gives curry its distinct bright yellow colour. Researchers believe it may play a key role in fighting several serious diseases associated with ageing.

Among many claims, a combined research team from the US, Finland and Hong Kong, as well as teams working in Italy, at the New York Medical College and at Oxford University and Churchill Hospital Research Institute claim that curcumin can fight some cancers and autoimmune diseases such as multiple sclerosis. The effects are thought to be due to the powerful antioxidant properties of curcumin and their action against free radical damage in a range of diseases, including brain ageing and neurodegenerative disorders. It also lowers bad cholesterol levels and protects the liver.

Many other spices have also been found to have important antioxidant and anti-inflammatory properties as well as acting as antivirals. It's no coincidence that more spices are used in hotter climates where their antibacterial action helps preserve food.

Capsicums
(which include chillies and paprika)

Excellent sources of beta carotene. There is also evidence to suggest they help speed up the metabolism and aid digestion and absorption of other nutrients.

Cumin, cardamom & coriander

Useful spices for flavour as well as their potent nutritional value. Try sprinkling them on stir-fried vegetables for extra taste or add cumin to steamed broccoli along with a little olive oil and soy sauce for a delicious and healthy vegetable dish.

Parsley

It is full of vitamin C (much more than oranges) and it stimulates the kidneys and acts as a diuretic so it's good for the digestion and getting rid of impurities and toxins. Full of vitamins A and C, iron, calcium and potassium. Use it as a:

- Breath-freshener after you've eaten garlic.
- Source of high levels of B12 to make your energy levels soar.

Cinnamon

As well as helping to control blood sugar levels, cinnamon has also been shown to reduce cholesterol levels, particularly harmful LDL cholesterol. Its antiseptic and anti-microbial properties make it helpful for sore throats and urinary tract and yeast infections.

Ginger

High in antioxidants and anti-inflammatories. It can improve circulation and combat nausea including travel sickness and the side-effects of chemotherapy. It's useful when it's cold outside or you feel under the weather. Add to soups and stir-fries, or make a warming infusion. Ginger boosts energy levels and stimulates the digestive system, helping it absorb nutrients. Simmer freshly grated ginger root in water and add lemon juice and honey to strengthen your liver and boost immunity.

Garlic

Antiviral, antifungal, antibiotic and anti-vampire. No, forget that last one. It's believed to have anti-ageing properties in Russia so maybe we should take a leaf out of their book. Like beetroot, it can help boost the intake of oxygen to cells which keeps the skin looking healthy.

Garlic is full of vitamin C which fights free radicals and boosts your immune system. It's also another powerful detoxifier and is packed full of selenium.

DID YOU KNOW?
Japanese mothers teach their children the importance of eating warming, stimulating foods like ginger and chilli in winter to stay warm and energized.

DID YOU KNOW?
Try sprinkling half a teaspoon of ground cinnamon on your coffee, tea or toast in the morning. It tastes delicious and it will help your heart. » According to a Norwegian study in the Journal of Nutrition, cinnamon is among the spices with the most anti-ageing, disease-fighting antioxidants.

And one you might not be expecting . . . Chocolate

Hurrah! Don't ever say I'm not good to you. Yes, good news it *is* an anti-ageing food. Bad news, you can't eat it by the bucket-load.

Research has shown that people who eat it one to three times a month cut their risk of early death by one third. This came from an eighty-year study of 7,800 Harvard graduates, which suggests that regular chocolate eaters (those who eat chocolates three times a week or more) live on average one extra year. Once-a-week chocolate eaters had a 15 per cent reduced risk of mortality compared with a 25 per cent reduced risk in the higher consumers. The reason? It's due to antioxidants called phenols found in chocolate; 40g (1½ oz) contains as much as a glass of red wine. But don't go mad, moderation at all times – chocolate contains mainly saturated fat which can raise blood cholesterol, increasing the risk of heart disease. Be careful not to eat too much as this stimulates insulin production which breaks down collagen and increases the wrinkle-effect on our skin.

DID YOU KNOW?
Chocolate contains phenylethylamine, the same chemical that floods your brain during orgasm. Cocoa solids contain health-giving polyphenols. So if you are going to treat yourself to one or two squares a day and no more, go for the rich, 70 per cent dark chocolate.

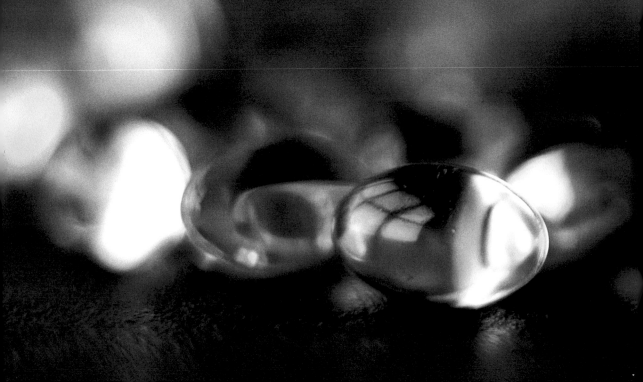

supplements

I'm a firm believer that it is always better to eat the nutrients you need in your food. It's the best way to make sure you are getting what you need and in the right combinations to ensure your body actually absorbs all the goodness.

However, there are times when you are particularly stressed, have been ill or just know you have been skimping on meals when supplements have a role to play in boosting nutrition. A number are particularly effective at holding back the worst signs of ageing, making you feel livelier and younger while at the same time preventing the formation of wrinkles and lines.

There are some combinations of supplements which can work well together, but generally I always recommend taking individual ones rather than multi-purpose multi-vitamins or minerals. That way you can target what you really need. I have deliberately not given RDAs as these vary so much for different products and brands. Also, individual requirements vary. I would always advise getting expert help. Just because many supplements are 'natural' does not mean they're not also very potent. Overdosing can be extremely serious and dangerous.

My top 20 anti-ageing supplements

1 Alpha lipoic acid

Alpha lipoic acid is one of the most powerful anti-ageing compounds and it is both antioxidant and anti-inflammatory. It is called the 'universal antioxidant' because it is soluble in fat and water, which means it can work inside cells as well as in the cell membranes. Our cells contain small amounts of this co-enzyme.

⋯⋗ It is necessary for the metabolism of energy from food and so boosts cellular energy.

⋯⋗ It helps balance glucose levels and improves insulin function.

⋯⋗ It's also an effective free-radical scavenger and helps to protect our DNA.

⋯⋗ Taking alpha lipoic acid improves the performance of a range of other antioxidants including vitamins C and E and glutathione, which is an antioxidant containing selenium found in nearly every cell in the body.

⋯⋗ It is claimed to be the best way to avoid the cross-linking glycation process that leads to ageing, brittle collagen and in the end sagging, wrinkled skin.

⋯⋗ Recent studies suggest alpha lipoic acid may also protect eyes.

⋯⋗ The co-enzyme is found in vegetables like broccoli but not in sufficient quantities for you to really notice the benefits.

IMPORTANT NOTE:
Before taking any supplements, or before radically changing your diet, you should always consult your doctor first, especially if you are taking any medication or have an underlying medical condition. Pregnant women should ALWAYS get medical advice before taking anything.

2 Carnitine

L-carnitine and acetyl-L-carnitine are two forms of the amino acid carnitine. The body normally converts L-carnitine which is produced in the liver into acetyl-L-carnitine. Levels in the body decrease after the age of 40.

L-carnitine

- Carries essential fatty acids to the cells and is vital for the production of energy from fat.
- By improving fat metabolism it can encourage weight loss.
- It guards against free radical damage.
- Extensive research shows L-carnitine to be effective for heart health, weight management, efficient exercise and improved brain function.
- Food sources include dairy products and meat.

Acetyl-L-carnitine

- Helps cells produce more energy.
- It can be classed as a 'brain food' as it can cross the brain-blood barrier.
- It improves thinking processes and memory.
- It is found throughout the central nervous system.
- Helps to restore and protect against ageing processes and nerve degeneration.
- Restores and improves skin health, helping it to look younger.
- When taken with L-carnitine, it seems to increase the rate of fat loss.
- There are no food sources for acetyl-L-carnitine.

DID YOU KNOW?
Bruce Ames, Professor of Molecular and Cell Biology at the University of California, Berkeley, studied the use of L-carnitine and alpha lipoic acid supplements together and believes they deliver a powerful attack on ageing cells. 'Each chemical solves a different problem,' he explains. 'The two together are better than either one alone.'

3 Co-enzyme Q10

This is another amino acid which is produced naturally by the body.

⋯⋗ A number of factors including age, illness, cholesterol-lowering drugs and poor nutrition can all hamper the body's ability to produce its own co-enzyme Q10 (also known as CoQ10).

⋯⋗ It has two important roles: it is an essential part of the mitochondria, or energy furnace of our cells, and an antioxidant.

⋯⋗ This means CoQ10 improves the rate and efficiency of energy production in our cells and protects them from free radical damage.

⋯⋗ It has been called a 'biomarker' of ageing because levels in the body correlate with ageing and age-related diseases.

⋯⋗ A number of studies have demonstrated the value of CoQ10 in helping heart failure and other degenerative heart diseases.

⋯⋗ It also relieves hypertension, decreased immunity and loss of muscle mass.

⋯⋗ It helps brain and nerve function and may benefit the skin.

⋯⋗ Main food sources are bony oily fish, like sardines, and peanuts, but only very small amounts are present.

4 DMAE

DMAE (or, to give it its full name, dimethylaminoethanol) is a neurotransmitter. It is found in small amounts in the brain and known for its brain-enhancing effects.

⋯⋗ It works to allow nerves to communicate with one another or with muscles.

⋯⋗ It is also an antioxidant which protects cell membranes.

⋯⋗ DMAE improves our thinking processes and increases alertness.

⋯⋗ It also helps alleviate mood swings and promotes feelings of calmness.

⋯⋗ As a neurotransmitter it increases muscle tone in the face and body.

⋯⋗ Its nutrient values can actually reverse skin sagging and drooping eyelids.

⋯⋗ DMAE is found in oily fish like salmon and anchovies.

5 Evening primrose oil

This oil has been around for such a long time that it is easy to overlook its benefits. A recent study in the *International Journal of Cosmetic Science* reported that taking six 500mg capsules of pure evening primrose oil a day stopped the effects of skin ageing in just three months.

⋯⟫ It is a very nourishing oil and a good source of the essential fatty acid GLA (or gamma linolenic acid).

⋯⟫ It is anti-inflammatory and very soothing.

⋯⟫ Its ability to inhibit bacterial growth means it is often used to treat eczema and psoriasis.

⋯⟫ The oil can be effective in easing PMS.

⋯⟫ The latest evidence from a research team at Northwestern University, Illinois, suggests the GLA in the oil may give added protection against breast cancer.

6 Glutamine

This is another amino acid which has a protective function. Like other amino acids, its levels in the body fall as a result of age or illness.

⋯⟫ It is found in proteins and is very important for metabolizing protein.

⋯⟫ It boosts energy and counters fatigue.

⋯⟫ It helps the gastrointestinal tract to heal and can treat some intestinal diseases.

⋯⟫ Glutamine supports the liver.

⋯⟫ It also prevents the breakdown of muscles and tissues and is useful for maintaining muscles. As a result it's particularly useful for athletes or anyone exercising.

⋯⟫ It helps strengthen the immune system.

⋯⟫ It balances blood sugar levels and can reduce cravings for sweets.

⋯⟫ Glutamine has been used effectively in the treatment of alcoholism and mild depression.

⋯⟫ Food sources include fish, poultry, beans and peas.

7 Grapeseed extract

Grapeseed extract belongs to a group of naturally occurring substances known as oligomeric proanthocyanidins. They are found in a wide variety of plants and foods and you can recognize their presence by the distinct deep red, purple and blue colours.

⇢ This is a very powerful antioxidant.

⇢ It helps to strengthen capillaries and the vascular system and may prevent varicose veins from developing.

⇢ It boosts the immune system.

⇢ It also works to repair connective tissue and so improves the strength of collagen and skin tone, preventing the formation of wrinkles and sagging.

⇢ Grapeseed extract can help control allergies.

⇢ When choosing a product look for dark-coloured red/purple capsules to make sure you are buying the most natural and best quality.

⇢ Take grapeseed extract at the same time as other vitamins as it works synergistically with them.

⇢ You will get a stronger antioxidant effect if the extract is taken with vitamin C or E.

⇢ Food sources include all deep red, purple and blue fruits and vegetables, for instance blueberries, blackberries, figs, cherries, beetroot, aubergines and red wine.

'It is important to distinguish between what is fashionable and good and what is fashionable and bad.' NIGELLA LAWSON

8 Hyaluronic acid

Hyaluronic acid is a wonderful anti-ager for the skin, literally moisturizing from the inside out and smoothing wrinkles in the process.

⋯⟶ Over time, hyaluronic acid is depleted in the body due to the natural ageing process and other environmental factors like pollutants and sunlight.

⋯⟶ Hyaluronic acid is present in every tissue in the body, including skin, eyes, cartilage, blood vessels and joints.

⋯⟶ It is a 'super moisturizer', holding 500 times its own weight in water.

⋯⟶ It is this moisturizing ability which makes it so important for youthful skin.

⋯⟶ It fills the spaces between collagen and elastin fibres in the connective tissue and makes it soft, smooth and elastic.

⋯⟶ Studies show that just two to four months of supplementation can act like an instant face lift on fine lines and wrinkles.

⋯⟶ Food sources include beans, pulses, sweet potatoes, some starchy root vegetables (see page 37) and chicken or meat broth.

9 Microfiltered whey protein

This is one of the purest and most easily absorbed forms of protein. After the age of 35 your digestive enzymes can begin to diminish and some people just don't digest protein very effectively, in particular anyone with Type A blood.

⋯⟶ Microfiltered whey proteins are complete proteins, supplying the essential amino acids required for good health, but they are digested very easily. They are low in fat and cholesterol with no lactose or starch. This makes them ideal for anyone with diabetes or heart problems.

⋯⟶ Research suggests they are antioxidant.

⋯⟶ It is also suggested they may improve immune function and have anti-cancer effects.

⋯⟶ The amino acids help to prevent skin sagging and ease stiff joints.

Minerals

Minerals are the building blocks for our body, vital for healthy skin, bones, teeth, muscles, nerves and tissues. They also work with enzymes to prompt all the biochemical reactions that are necessary for our bodies to function. All are important but several have a special role in anti-ageing.

10 Chromium

⋯⇥ Chromium is important in the metabolism of carbohydrates and fats.
⋯⇥ It helps regulate and balance blood sugar levels.
⋯⇥ As a result it can help weight loss.
⋯⇥ It is also needed for insulin to function properly.
⋯⇥ There is some evidence that it may be useful in the treatment of diabetes.
⋯⇥ Chromium also helps build lean muscle tissue.
⋯⇥ It can lower cholesterol levels.
⋯⇥ It is absorbed best if taken with vitamin C.
⋯⇥ Chromium polynicotinate is the recommended form of the supplement (there have been safety concerns about chromium picolinate damaging the DNA in cells which could lead to cancer).
⋯⇥ Food sources include calves' liver and brewer's yeast.

11 Calcium

⋯⇥ Calcium gives strength to bones and teeth and guards against the loss of bone density.
⋯⇥ A good supply of calcium is essential throughout our lives.
⋯⇥ If anything, it becomes even more important for women as they approach menopause when they need extra calcium to guard against osteoporosis.
⋯⇥ Calcium can relieve symptoms of PMS.
⋯⇥ It is important for muscle contraction and can prevent muscle cramp.
⋯⇥ It reduces cholesterol levels and can lower blood pressure.
⋯⇥ It also improves nerve function.
⋯⇥ Calcium helps the absorption of nutrients.
⋯⇥ Deficiencies can lead to osteoporosis and rickets.
⋯⇥ There are two types of calcium supplement – chelated forms are absorbed more easily by the body but the second type, calcium carbonate, is cheaper.
⋯⇥ Food sources include dairy products, oily bony fish like sardines, wheatgerm, leafy green vegetables, nuts and seeds.

12 Magnesium

- It is found in trace amounts in the body.
- Magnesium regulates blood pressure and blood sugar levels.
- It is also important for nerve function.
- It helps to maintain muscles, nerves and bones.
- Improves muscle and therefore skin tone.
- It also relieves the negative ageing effects of stress on the body.
- The mineral is used to metabolize energy and protein synthesis.
- Some recent research suggests a magnesium deficiency may play a role in causing migraine headaches.
- Food sources include oatmeal, avocados, almonds and soya beans.
- Cooking dissolves magnesium, so more than half can be lost from food sources.

13 Selenium

- This is an essential dietary mineral but it is toxic at higher doses, so always follow the dosage instructions on the packaging.
- Selenium activates an enzyme called glutathione peroxidase which may protect the body from cancer.
- It is an important antioxidant, protecting cells against the damaging effects of free radicals.
- It also has antifungal properties.
- Selenium may help the body neutralize the effects of toxins like mercury.
- It is important for heart function and a healthy immune system.
- Food sources include brazil nuts, liver, garlic, poultry and fish.

14 Omega essential fatty acids and fish oil

Essential fatty acids are vital for healthy nutrition. They protect the heart, lower cholesterol levels, blood pressure and reduce the chance of blood clots. It is even thought they can protect against some cancers. These fats promote healthy skin, bones, tissues and hair – in a word, they are essential for health and to hold back the signs of ageing. For more on the differences between Omega-3, -6 and -9 see pages 45–49.

DID YOU KNOW?
It is estimated that over 85 per cent of people in the Western world are deficient in Omega-3 fatty acids, while most get too much Omega-6.

···⟩ In most cases the western diet is high in Omega-6 but lacking in Omega-3.

···⟩ Omega-3 is vital for the body to use Omega-6 properly.

···⟩ Omega-3 reduces inflammation in the body which is a major cause of ageing.

···⟩ Omega-3 is particularly effective against leukotrines which are the chemicals produced by free radicals which can cause skin problems and allergies.

···⟩ Omega-3 is especially important in lowering harmful LDL cholesterol levels and triglycerides and increasing good HDL cholesterol levels.

···⟩ It lowers blood pressure and improves the health of your heart.

···⟩ It has also been shown to relieve stiff joints and rheumatoid arthritis.

···⟩ Fish oil is the best source of Omega-3 because it contains the most beneficial of the fatty acids – EPA and DHA – but it is important to choose the right fish oil.

Choose a fish oil that states it is:

···⟩ High in Omega-3 containing the essential fatty acids DHA and EPA.

···⟩ Purified to the highest standards to ensure there are no detectable levels of mercury, cadmium, lead, PCBs and other contaminants.

···⟩ Free from chemical modification and unprocessed.

Fish pollution

Fish of all varieties from all water sources are now showing dangerously high levels of the tasteless but highly toxic metal, mercury, as well as other pollutants. So unless you are certain the fish oil you are taking has been independently tested and shown to be free of toxins, I would advise you to avoid it. That said, I recommend fish oil as a supplement to almost everyone's diet – from child to senior citizen and every age in between.

Oil quality

The processing and packaging of the fish oil are crucial in determining its quality. Low-quality oils may be quite unstable as well as containing significant levels of toxins. High-quality oils are stabilized with adequate amounts of vitamin E and are packaged to protect them from light and oxygen. The best choice is oil made from deep-water ocean fish. These fish tend to have the highest content of EPA and DHA to ensure their body fat stays supple in the icy cold waters.

Some very recent research carried out at the University of Minnesota found that emulsified fish oils are much better absorbed than the straight oils in gelatine capsules.

Sources of fish oil

Cod liver oil and fish oils are not the same. Cod liver oil is extracted from cod liver and is an excellent source of vitamins A and D. Fish oils are extracted from the tissues (flesh) of fatty fish like salmon and herring and are good sources of the essential fatty acids EPA and DHA. Fish oils contain very little vitamin A and D, but cod liver oil does contain some EPA and DHA. However, you would probably exceed the recommended safe daily intake of vitamins A and D if you were to try to obtain beneficial amounts of EPA and DHA from cod liver oil.

Supplementing with fish oils has been found to be safe and no significant adverse effects have been reported in hundreds of clinical trials. Fish oil supplements do, however, lower blood concentrations of vitamin E so it is a good idea to take extra vitamin E when adding fish oils to your diet.

A clinical trial carried out by the US Department of Agriculture found that taking 200mg per day of synthetic vitamin E (equivalent to about 100iu of natural alpha-tocopherol or vitamin E) is enough to make up for this and many fish oils also contain added vitamin E.

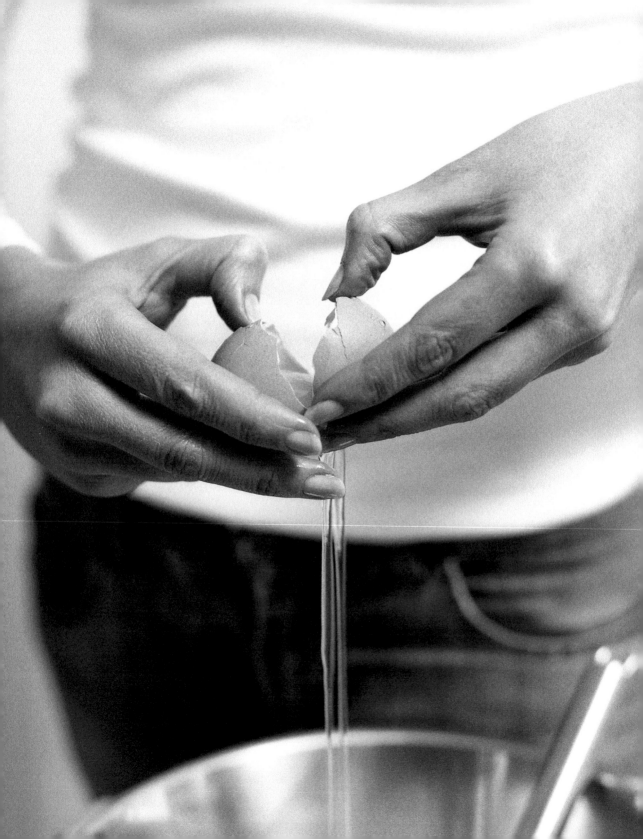

15 Zinc

···> Zinc is important for the production of enzymes needed for cell division and repair.

···> It helps the immune system to function properly and speeds healing of wounds.

···> It also maintains supple, healthy collagen and skin.

···> It boosts metabolism and energy levels.

···> Zinc is essential for proper nutrition, improving digestion, taste and smell.

···> It is also important in reproduction, growth and the control of diabetes.

···> Zinc neutralizes free radicals and is vital for the body to function properly.

···> A deficiency can cause hair loss.

···> Food sources include eggs, poultry, oatmeal, mushrooms, fish and brazil nuts.

16 Rosehip oil

Cold-pressed rosehip oil is a wonderful, natural anti-ager. It can be used topically to soothe, rejuvenate, moisturize and repair damaged skin. But it works just as effectively taken as a supplement.

···> The essential fatty acids it contains help repair cell membranes.

···> The prostaglandins it triggers support the immune system, balance moisture levels and control inflammation.

···> The oil contains tretinoin (a derivative of retinol, or vitamin A), which nourishes and helps rebuild skin tissue.

···> It can reduce scarring and fine lines.

···> Rosehip oil also contains lycopene, the powerful antioxidant that is found in tomatoes. Lycopene prevents free radical damage and helps protect against the worst effects of the sun.

···> Like evening primrose oil, rosehip oil may also relieve some symptoms of PMS.

Vitamins

Vitamins are vital for the normal functioning of our bodies, necessary for growth, energy and general well-being. They help to regulate the metabolism converting carbohydrates and fats into energy.
It is important to remember that vitamin supplements are not a replacement for food and they cannot be properly absorbed without food which is why the usual advice is to take them with a meal.

···⟩ Vitamins are either fat or water soluble.

···⟩ Vitamins A, D and E are fat soluble which means they are stored in the liver and so levels can build up and become toxic to the body.

···⟩ Vitamins B and C are water soluble which means they are not stored by the body and can be used up relatively quickly. Any excess is lost in urine.

17 Vitamin A

···⟩ It helps cells to reproduce properly and can guard against cancerous changes in cells.

···⟩ It helps healthy growth and bone development.

···⟩ Vitamin A is essential for healthy vision and particularly important for night vision.

···⟩ It boosts the immune system and speeds wound healing.

···⟩ Vitamin A improves the skin's elasticity, helping to keep skin moisturized, smooth, supple and youthful.

···⟩ It protects mucus membranes in the mouth, nose and airways which reduce our susceptibility to infection and protect against pollution.

···⟩ A lack of vitamin A can lead to dry, rough skin and eye problems.

···⟩ As well as being found in meat, poultry, dairy products and fish, vitamin A is also found as carotene (its precurser) in fruit and vegetables including spinach, watercress, apricots, peaches and cantaloupe melon.

···⟩ Vitamin A supplements are not recommended at all for pregnant women.

18 B group vitamins

···⟩ B group vitamins are a complex of important vitamins including B1, B2, B6, B12, pantothenic acid (B5) and folic acid (B9).

···⟩ They work as co-enzymes alongside one another to perform essential body processes.

···⟩ They are vital for a healthy brain, nerves and skin and form the basis of any anti-ageing programme.

···⟩ These vitamins are essential for metabolizing energy from food.

···⟩ They maintain healthy skin, hair and nails and can prevent skin problems.

···⟩ B vitamins support the immune system.

···⟩ They are also responsible for a healthy nervous system and help the body cope with stress.

···⟩ B vitamins boost energy and combat fatigue, mood swings and insomnia.

···⟩ A B12 deficiency can lead to anaemia as it is important in the formation of red blood cells.

···⟩ The B group also improve liver health.

···⟩ These vitamins are anti-inflammatory.

···⟩ They promote brain function.

···⟩ They strengthen bones and muscles.

···⟩ They are also useful for relieving PMT.

···⟩ Food sources include yeast, whole grains, nuts including almonds and walnuts, chickpeas, lentils, chicken, fish, eggs, parsnips, spinach and avocados.

'Don't worry about middle age. You'll outgrow it.' LAURENCE J PETER

19 Vitamin C

- This is probably the most important antioxidant anti-ageing substance you can take.
- It is one of the best defenders against free radical damage.
- Vitamin C is vital for the immune system and builds a resistance to infection.
- It helps wounds and scar tissue heal.
- It maintains healthy bones, teeth and gums.
- It strengthens blood vessels.
- Vitamin C is also essential for the proper absorption of a range of nutrients including iron.
- It is also important for neurotransmitters to function properly.
- In terms of the obvious signs of ageing, vitamin C is responsible for the production of collagen and so maintains muscle tone and prevents the development of wrinkles and lines.
- It also helps the skin to repair itself and slows the formation of melanin which means it inhibits the development of age or sun spots.
- Food sources of vitamin C include strawberries, kiwi fruit, apricots, citrus fruits, tomatoes, broccoli and peppers.

Slow-release vitamin C

As well as the standard L-ascorbic acid form of vitamin C, there is now a slow-release form. Vitamin C is not stored and is constantly washed from the body. In fact, it usually remains for only a few hours. Because it needs to be regularly supplemented through diet to replace the loss, the idea behind the slow-release form is to give your body a constant, usable supply of the vitamin.

Many nutritionists are in favour but there is disagreement. Some would argue that the body does not need a constant supply and that in some cases it may even be harmful. There is also some question about whether time-release vitamins in general are absorbed less efficiently.

20 Vitamin E

- Vitamin E belongs to a group called tocopherols.
- It is a potent antioxidant and one of the best known.
- It prevents cell damage which may lead to cancer.
- It helps in the formation of red blood cells and in the utilization of vitamin K – responsible for blood clotting.
- Vitamin E lowers harmful LDL cholesterol levels and reduces the risk of heart disease and stroke.
- It can prevent blood clots and reduce blood pressure.
- This vitamin protects cell membranes and other 'oily' body structures, including the skin.
- Vitamin E has been called nature's healer and it speeds wound healing and prevents scarring, actually helping the regeneration of scarred skin.
- This vitamin also boosts the immune system.
- Vitamin E is thought to protect against cataracts.
- It has also been shown to be useful for Alzheimers sufferers.
- As with other vitamins, a complete lack of vitamin E in the diet is fatal, but the amount needed for basic health is very small.
- Food sources include whole grains, nuts and seeds.

Vitamin E supplements

It used to be true that synthetic forms were not very effective. Now more is understood about the formulation of the vitamin and if it is properly produced, a supplement can be very effective if taken with food.

Look out for brands where the manufacturer clearly states that the supplement contains only the D form of the vitamin. This makes it much closer in composition to the natural vitamin.

Other supplements

As well as the 20 super supplements detailed on the previous pages there are a few others which can be useful in the fight against ageing.

To support your liver

Milk thistle

⋯⋗ Milk thistle is a common roadside plant, related to the artichoke which has been used as a tonic since Roman times. It is a powerful antioxidant and in particular it works to support the liver, helping it flush out toxins and repair damaged cells.

⋯⋗ The liver is vital as a filter for blood, processing and removing waste products. For our body to function properly and cope with everything we throw at it, the liver must work efficiently. In fact this is key if we are to remain feeling and looking healthy and youthful.

⋯⋗ Liver spots are another name for the age spots which can appear on ageing skin. Often they are the result of sun damage but they can also be a sign of a sluggish liver. If so, taking a milk thistle supplement will help.

For brain power

Ginkgo biloba

⋯⋗ This is one of the best-selling herbal products in the world and has been used for over 5000 years in Asia to treat heart and lung problems. Recently US researchers have identified the active flavonoids ginkgo contains which work to increase blood circulation to the brain and other organs.

⋯⋗ As well as helping circulatory problems and strengthening arteries it also improves memory and mental performance and it is now being researched for its possible role in combating a range of problems, including senility, forgetfulness, headaches and Alzheimer's. The powerful antioxidants it contains can maintain cells and defend the body against free radicals.

Ginseng

⋯⋗ This is the dried root of one of several species of herbs. There are several different types including Asian (also called Panax, Chinese or Korean) and American which is closely related to it. Siberian ginseng is different.

⋯⋗ Ginseng is widely used in the US to improve energy and vitality and is thought to be particularly helpful in times of stress. It's thought to stimulate the immune system and may give protection against colds and flu. When taken with ginkgo biloba, it's particularly effective in improving memory.

Buying supplements

⋯⋗ Most of the supplements mentioned here should be readily available from good health stores and complementary medicine pharmacies.

⋯⋗ If you have difficulty sourcing anything, there are several good sites online. Victoria Health (www.victoriahealth.com) is one of the best, with up-to-date information on the latest news and developments as well as an easy-to-use search facility where you can buy all of these products. Also, see the directory at the end of the book.

'Just as we can alter the lifespan of a car by how well or badly we drive and maintain it, we alter the ageing of our body by how well or badly we take care of it.'

DR TOM KIRKWOOD, UK LONGEVITY EXPERT

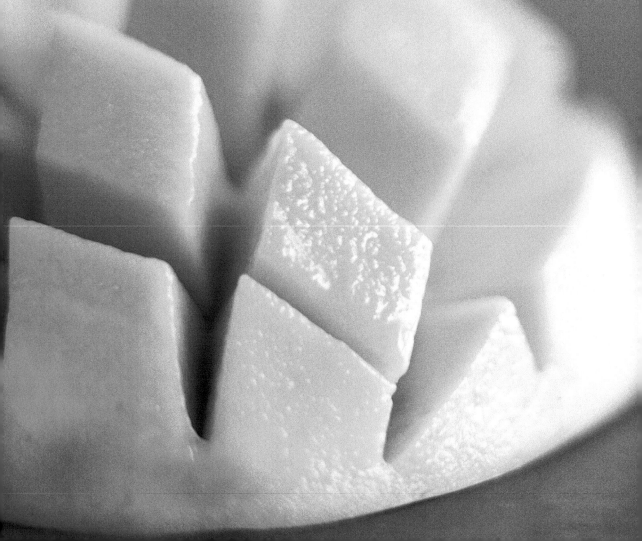

CHAPTER FIVE

habits, hormones, moods and foods

So many of my happiest memories have a common theme – eating. Don't get me wrong, I'm not obsessed with what I eat – honestly, it's quite the opposite! Whether I'm remembering a family get-together or friends meeting up, a meal has usually been involved – from a full-blown banquet to a simple supper in my mum's kitchen. And that's probably true for you too. A huge part of our lives is based around food, yet half of us seem to be eating ourselves into an early grave, while the other half are locked into the latest faddy diet – all of which is incredibly ageing. What happened to sitting down and enjoying a meal that looks good, tastes great and knocks years off at the same time?

The more extreme you are (eating too much or too little, depriving yourself of carbs, avoiding fats...), the less balance there is in your diet, which is ultimately ageing. As far as I'm concerned, dieting doesn't work; it is not the answer to looking and feeling younger. Having a balanced diet – a completely different thing from dieting – does. This book is about developing habits that work for you and become so much part of your life that you don't even think about them. An anti-ageing diet isn't about depriving yourself. My message for eating yourself younger is simple: keep it balanced, all things in moderation and enjoy your food.

Why do we eat?

Simple question really, but lots of different answers. Mainly, we eat because we get hungry and we need food and water to keep us alive. The vitamins and minerals give us the energy to keep going, to repair the wear and tear on our minds and bodies. With the right nutrients, we can also keep ourselves feeling great and looking younger.

The food bank

Somebody once described our energy requirements as a bit like having a bank account. When we eat, we make deposits in our energy bank. We make withdrawals when our body expends energy. And we use up energy whatever we're doing – getting up in the morning, cleaning our teeth, walking to the bus, sitting at our desk . . . The trick, like running your finances efficiently, is to achieve the right balance between the withdrawals and deposits.

We also eat when we're:

- ⋯⋗ Lonely
- ⋯⋗ Depressed and bored
- ⋯⋗ Stressed out
- ⋯⋗ Bereaved
- ⋯⋗ Sexually frustrated
- ⋯⋗ Angry

'If I'd known I was going to live so long, I'd have taken better care of myself.' LEON ELDRED

If you're lonely – you tend to go for filling, comfort foods, heavy on the carbohydrates. Carbs give an energy boost and increase the production of serotonin, so eating carbohydrate-rich foods can make you feel a bit better. No bad thing but be careful not to over-indulge because the excess sugar will be stored as fat and have an ageing effect on your skin.

If you're depressed – studies found people reach for stimulants like coffee with sugar. Coffee gives an immediate hit, but is bad news in the long run. If you are depressed you are often low in vitamin B6, so include lots of green leafy vegetables in your diet to redress the balance and perk yourself up.

If you're stressed – we reach for salty foods because our adrenaline glands send out signals demanding more salt. But too much salt can raise blood pressure which, again, has an ageing effect on the body (see page 253 for tips on how to eat when feeling stressed).

If you've suffered a loss – when we lose someone or a relationship breaks up, comfort food is top of the list. Again, the serotonin has the feel-good factor but comfort food can be full of fat and sugar (yes, you know it – ageing). Go for healthy serotonin-rich foods (a banana smoothie is ideal).

If you're sexually frustrated – believe it or not, crunchy foods like crackers or toast are the popular choice here. Zinc, found in oily fish, seafood and pumpkin, is a great libido-booster (and essential for the production of collagen). Perhaps to be avoided if there's no opportunity for – how can I put it delicately – scratching an itch!

If you're angry – again, chewy, crunchy food helps relieve feelings of anger. It's sort of the food alternative to grinding your teeth. Go for the healthy option if you feel a bit wound up – carrots are full of protective anti-ageing antioxidants and give a satisfying crunch at the same time.

DID YOU KNOW?
In a survey conducted by the British Dietetic Association, a third of people questioned said they ended up heavier than their original weight only weeks after dieting. » Researchers at Tufts University, Massachusetts, found that the more variety there is in your diet, the more likely you are to lose weight. » A Hummer H2 could be driven around the world 244 times on the excess calories Americans consume each year (*Harpers* magazine).

'To eat well in England you should have breakfast three times a day.'

W SOMERSET MAUGHAM

How often to eat

I eat three times a day and I don't snack between meals. Snacking can send your blood sugar levels on a rollercoaster ride which ultimately plays havoc with your body, your looks and your temperament. If you really can't do without, eat five or six small meals a day (see Food Plans, page 283, for some healthy ideas).

Loads of people still skip breakfast, only eat a very light lunch and have their largest meal of the day in the evening. Why? Do you think you're keeping your calorie count down and being healthy? Don't be fooled; you're only setting yourself up for a major snack attack in the afternoon and a huge dinner in the evening. If you want to look younger and feel great, breakfast is the most important meal of the day. *Don't miss it*. Turn to page 240 for some brilliant breakfasts.

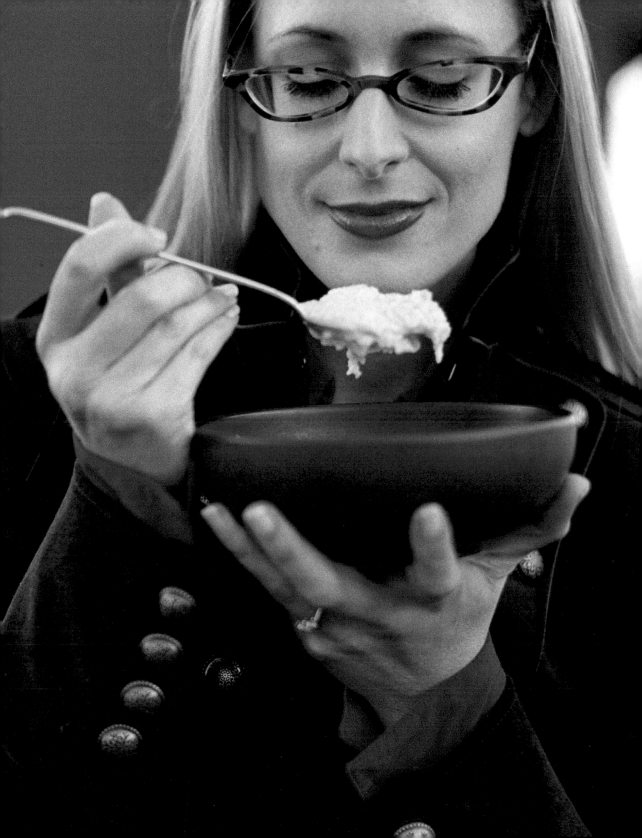

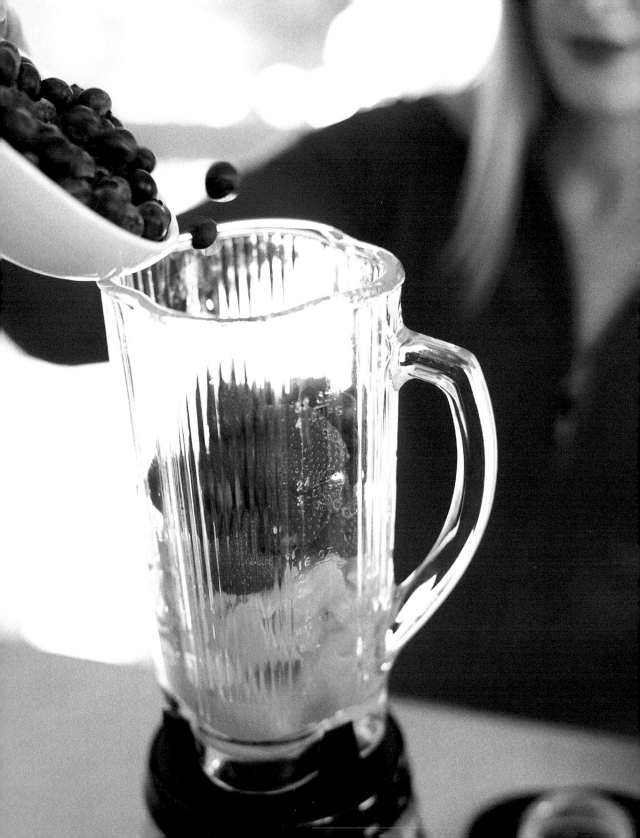

Avoiding the sugar rush

If your blood sugar levels have gone haywire, then your body craves a sugar hit. Sugar is one of the most damaging and ageing foods on our bodies. It destroys collagen which we need to hold wrinkles at bay and it ruins your digestion which leads to bloating, cramp, sluggishness and headaches. Sugar, like salt, is hidden in loads of food nowadays so you keep an eye on what you are eating. A tell-tale sign that you've taken too much sugar on board is if you feel sleepy after a meal. To avoid sugar:

···⟩ Avoid processed foods (biscuits, crisps, cakes, chocolates, pasta, bread).
···⟩ Remember sugar isn't just found in 'sweet' foods; even white flour turns into glucose really quickly.
···⟩ Cut back on alcohol.
···⟩ Choose foods that keep your blood sugar levels on an even keel.

In addition:
···⟩ Reduce the amount of saturated fat; use monounsaturated and polyunsaturated fat (pages 79–81 for fat facts).
···⟩ Fibre is good for you so opt for foods that contain whole grains or soluble fibre – oats, lentils, fruit (page 86 for fibre facts).
···⟩ Eat fish regularly, at least twice a week. In particular, oily fish such as salmon (see page 122 for the low-down on oily fish).
···⟩ Drink more water. I've waxed lyrical many times on how brilliant water is. Quite simply this is the best beauty aid in the world. It doesn't have to cost you anything, you can get hold of it any time of the day and it does wonders for your skin. What more can I say?

DID YOU KNOW?
If you find it difficult to drink 2 litres of water a day, do what I do – drink four small 500ml bottles. It seems more manageable.

Working with your metabolism

Your metabolism, or the rate at which your body burns calories, is like an engine; the more often you give it fuel, the better it works (for an in-depth look at the metabolism, see pages 68–72).

When you deprive your body of food:

⋯⋗ Your metabolism slows down to hang on to energy to preserve it.

⋯⋗ A slowed metabolism makes it much more difficult to lose weight and much easier to gain weight.

⋯⋗ An irregular eating pattern (not consistent in calorie and nutrient intake) will lead to a more rapid loss of muscle because the body is forced to take its energy from elsewhere.

⋯⋗ Muscle loss is ageing.

DID YOU KNOW?
Research shows that we are full of self-control after a good night's sleep, but that tends to decline as the day goes on. » A high-fat diet can increase your appetite for even more fatty food. Eating fatty food can prevent your brain from being able to tell when you're full. A Penn State University study found that rats fed on a long-term high-fat diet were less sensitive to the 'stop eating' hormone – yes, it does exist – cholecystokinin – and ate as much as 40 per cent more snacks than rats on a low-fat diet.

DID YOU KNOW?
It takes 20 minutes for the stretch receptors in your stomach lining to send a message to your brain registering food.

⋯⟩ Never, ever skip breakfast. It gives your metabolism an instant boost.

⋯⟩ Eat to keep your energy up and your blood sugar levels on an even keel. You'll avoid overloading your system and shouldn't feel hungry which can affect performance. The aim is to keep a balance in how you eat and what you eat.

⋯⟩ Chew each mouthful slowly; you release more nutrients this way and it helps to digest food properly. Eating slowly helps you feel full faster and will help to prevent overeating. If you eat too quickly, your stomach doesn't register that it's full until it's too late.

⋯⟩ Replace your normal dinner plates (which are usually 28–33cm/11–13in in diameter) with smaller plates. Your portion sizes have to go down but your plates still look full.

⋯⟩ Try not to eat on the run. Sitting down to a meal means you enjoy your food more and you avoid upsetting your digestion. A study by the University of Minnesota has found that eating at the table with the family has lots of other benefits – such as improved communication in the family. Children who ate with their families did better at school and were less likely to be depressed.

⋯⟩ Control your alcohol intake – alcohol is full of empty calories and it doesn't do much for your self-control either. Studies have shown that people who drink while they eat tend to eat more than those who don't.

⋯⟩ Watch out for the snack attack cues and change your behaviour round them – remove forms of temptation (like nibbling on something unsuitable when you're watching television – take up knitting or do the ironing).

⋯⟩ Go to bed early. People who don't have enough sleep have lower levels of leptin, a hormone that tells your brain you're full, and higher levels of ghrelin, a hormone that triggers hunger.

DID YOU KNOW?
A recent survey conducted by the French Government's Committee for Health Education (CFES) found that: 76 per cent of the French population eat meals they have prepared at home. » The favourite place to eat both lunch and dinner is in the home. » 75 per cent eat at the family table.

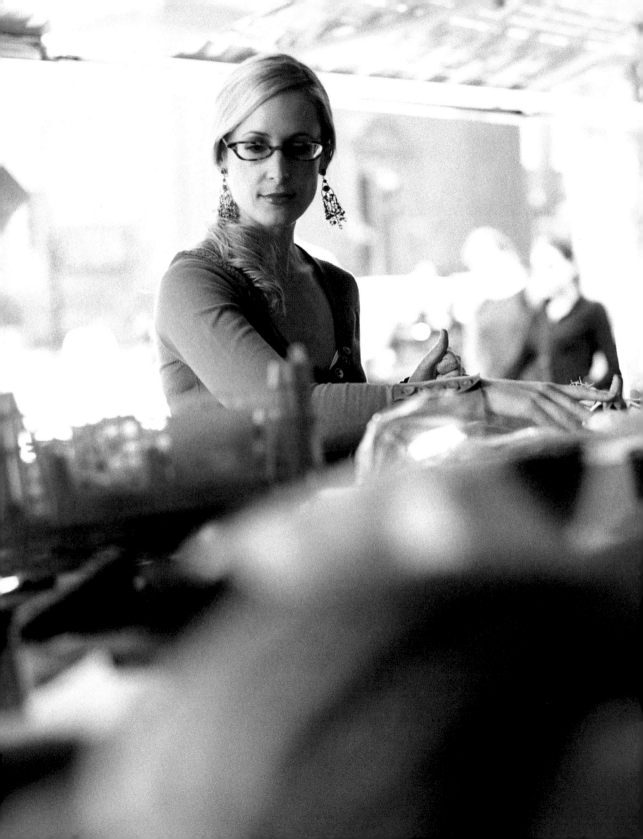

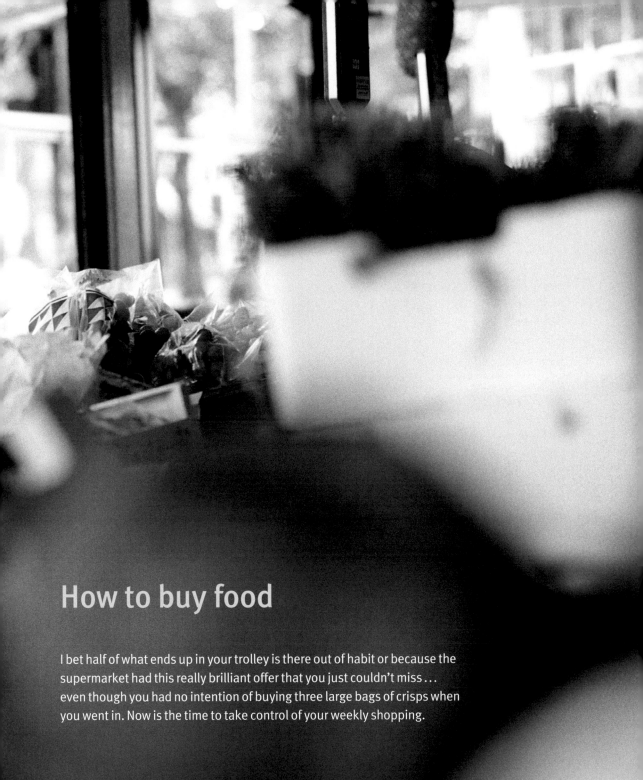

How to buy food

I bet half of what ends up in your trolley is there out of habit or because the supermarket had this really brilliant offer that you just couldn't miss ... even though you had no intention of buying three large bags of crisps when you went in. Now is the time to take control of your weekly shopping.

Sensible shopping

⋯⋗ Eat before you go shopping – then you're less likely to buy quick-fix ageing snacks.

⋯⋗ Write a list and stick to it. A big part of managing a healthy, anti-ageing diet is planning ahead. That means buying the right kind of food and not being tempted by unsuitable bargains and offers as you trail round the supermarket.

⋯⋗ Shop for fruit and vegetables first. The government recommends that we eat *at least* five portions of fruit and vegetables a day and they really are full of key anti-ageing nutrients. But the reality is that we eat fewer than three. Not keen on apples and cauliflower? You've got a huge range to choose from (see pages 236–237 to get an idea of some fab fruits and veg).

⋯⋗ Don't be tempted to buy ready meals. It really is so much better for you (and kinder on your purse) to make meals from scratch yourself. Ready meals are full of preservatives, salt and sugar – all of which do nothing to hold back the years. Around 80 per cent of our salt intake comes from processed and ready-made food. Make double the amount of soups, stews and casseroles and freeze the surplus.

⋯⋗ The fresher the fruit and veg, the better. The longer they are exposed to light and air, the more valuable, rejuvenating nutrients are lost. Some fruit and veg, stored at normal room temperature for a week, can lose up to 50 per cent of their natural vitamins.

⋯⋗ Fresh, however, is not the only option: frozen and canned foods are still full of vital minerals and vitamins (British Nutrition Foundation). As soon as they are picked, they are frozen or canned. Canned food does lose some of its important nutrients during the canning process but, if buying canned guava or pineapple is the only way you can get your hands on the fruit, then that's so much better than not getting it at all. Go for food that is stored in water rather than brine or syrup.

⋯⋗ Have a good read ... of the labels. They are full of important information that can help you make the sensible choice.

⋯⋗ Let your fingers do the walking – use the internet to do your weekly shopping. Most major supermarkets offer home delivery and you can control what you choose from the comfort of your own home.

⋯⟩ Buy seasonally and locally wherever possible – the food is fresh, full of wrinkle-busting nutrients and hasn't clocked up thousands of air miles getting to you. Farmers' markets are a great place to get locally produced, good food.

⋯⟩ Organic food comes free from preservatives, GM-modification and generally hasn't been mucked about with (see page 208 for more information on buying and eating organic food). Yes, it is more expensive than the non-organic equivalent but the taste and health benefits are worth putting it on your shopping list, even if only as a treat now and again.

DID YOU KNOW?
If a 200g bag of salad leaves costs about £1 and a whole 600g lettuce about 60p, that means there's a 500 per cent mark-up on the bag of salad. Buy a whole lettuce and wash and shred it at home, as and when you need it. It's a cheaper and healthier option. » Only 1 in 600 school lunch boxes contain a salad. » We bought less fruit and veg in 2003–4 than in the previous year; however, we consumed 9 per cent more alcohol (Dept of Environment, Food & Rural Affairs 2005). » A survey showed that a third of men were responsible for the main supermarket shop; over half admitted that their wife/partner wrote the list; 59 per cent did not stick to the list; 17 per cent said this caused rows.

'I eat to be healthy now, rather than to be thin.' GERI HALLIWELL

How to cook

How you cook food has as much impact on an anti-ageing diet as what food you buy. If you change the way you cook, you don't always have to cut out the kind of foods that you enjoy. Certain methods of cooking can preserve more vitamins and minerals in the food and help the body absorb more nutrients which we need to keep wrinkles at bay; while not every food is best eaten raw. For example:

Tomatoes – full of vitamin C when uncooked. However, cooking increases the levels of the phytochemical, lycopene. A small amount of fat with cooked tomato helps the body absorb more lycopene and beta carotene which are both powerful anti-ageing antioxidants.

Carrots – can be eaten raw, but actually are better for us when cooked. The cooking breaks down the tough cell walls so that it's easier for the body to use the beta carotene. Again, a small amount of fat increases the absorption of the beta carotene.

'Eating is not merely a material pleasure. Eating well gives a spectacular joy to life and contributes immensely to goodwill and happy companionship. It is of great importance to the morale.'

ELSA SCHIAPARELLI, ITALIAN DESIGNER

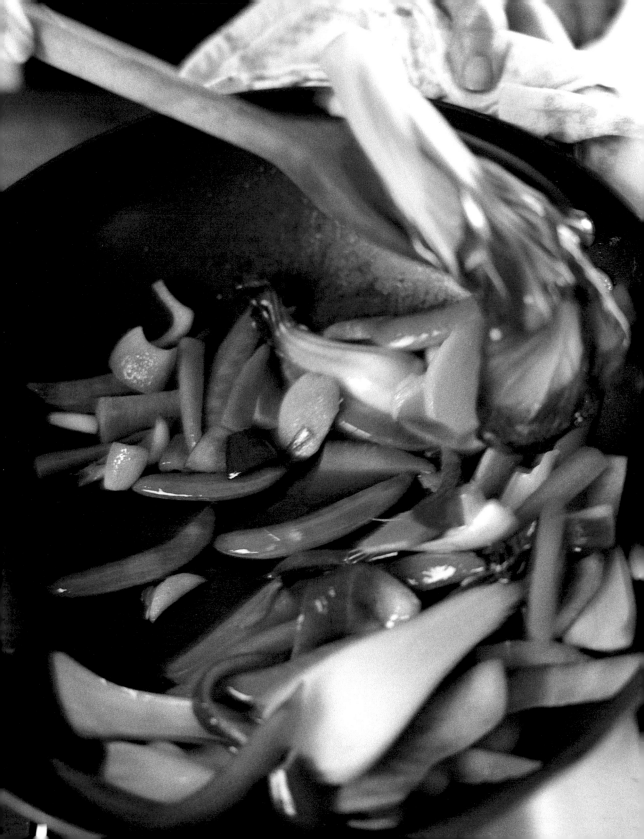

Cooking methods

The way you cook can be just as important as what you actually cook.

Steaming
This is ideal for fish and vegetables because you keep the maximum amount of nutrients and preserve the texture and taste.

Grilling
Very little fat is needed; ideal for lean meat and fish. Food cooks quickly so taste and nutrients are preserved.

Stir-frying
Food is cooked quickly in a wok over a high heat. Very little fat is needed. Again, fewer nutrients are lost this way than in other forms of cooking.

Microwaving
Microwaving with a little water for a short while preserves more vitamins and minerals.

Barbecuing
Finally, a quick word about barbecuing. In my native South Africa, it's practically the national way to cook. Many people think it's a very healthy form of cooking because you use very little fat to cook with. However, too much charcoal-barbecued meat can interfere with healthy liver function. Barbecued food also produces acrylamide which is known to be carcinogenic. I'm not saying don't ever barbecue again … just enjoy it as a treat now and again.

> **FACT FILE**
> Rather than use butter or lard in your cooking, opt for healthy oils such as olive and flax (see pages 79–80). » Try to keep food whole as much as possible. You can lose vitamins by chopping food up. » See page 305 for a list of store cupboard standbys.

Eating for sleep

Sleep is almost as important as food for helping you to look younger and feel great. It's also the time when your body sets about serious repair and maintenance work. Quite simply, if you don't get enough sleep this repair work won't happen, which is a health and ageing disaster. Sleep reduces the ageing effects of cortisol and increases the production of anti-ageing growth hormones.

The older we get, the longer it takes us to get to sleep and the less we need of it. Whether you can exist happily on six hours a night or, like me, need a full eight hours, what you eat and drink will have a major impact on the quality of your sleep.

The secret of a good night's sleep

⋯⋗ Have a glass of warm milk before bed – milk contains one of the eight essential amino acids, tryptophan, which helps relax you and bring on sleep. Tryptophan is an essential amino acid and a precursor of the hormone, serotonin, which controls the sleep cycle.

⋯⋗ Serotonin is a neurotransmitter. The yin to adrenaline's yang. It calms us down and reduces brain activity – ideal for dropping off to sleep. Carbohydrate-rich foods (like potatoes, pasta and bread) stimulate the body to produce the sleep-inducing serotonin hormones. Low sugar levels can affect our sleep; serotonin regulates sugar levels in the body.

⋯⋗ Carbohydrates also produce glucose which our brains need for refuelling overnight.

⋯⋗ If you really do need a late-night snack, a bowl of cornflakes with milk raises serotonin levels.

⋯⋗ High-protein meals will also keep you satisfied for longer and avoid cravings for midnight munchies. A seared tuna steak with green vegetables or, even better, a lettuce salad is ideal.

⋯⋗ You could also opt for turkey, tuna, figs, bananas, avocados, walnuts or yogurt (though not all together!) as they also contain tryptophan.

- Calcium and magnesium have a naturally tranquillizing effect; they're found in seeds, nuts and green leafy vegetables.

- Chamomile or valerian tea are great relaxers.

- Lettuce contains tryptophan. Lettuce also contains lactones, a natural sedative – remember the baby rabbits slumbering soundly after eating lettuce in Beatrix Potter's *Tale of the Flopsy Bunnies*?

- Melatonin, which helps regulate sleep, is also found in bananas, tomatoes, sweetcorn and rice.

- Don't eat too late at night. Try to allow at least two hours before you go to bed.

- You don't want to go to bed hungry as low blood sugar levels will stop your body producing sufficient sleep-promoting hormones.

DID YOU KNOW?
Elvis Presley's favourite snack, a peanut-butter and banana sandwich, will help you to sleep well at night thanks to the high levels of the amino acid, tryptophan.

Avoid:

- Caffeine which is found in coffee, tea and chocolate, so a late-night cocoa isn't the best way to get off to sleep.

- Sugar gives a rush of energy which is the last thing you need before trying to get to sleep. Rising blood sugar levels reduce the amount of growth-hormone production; this hormone is vital for repairing and renewing body cells. It's mainly produced during the first 90 minutes of sleep.

- Alcohol – it may make you drowsy at first and help you to drop off to sleep. But, a few hours later, it produces a burst of norepinephrine, a hormone that can jolt you awake in the wee small hours.

- Curries contain too many stimulants such as garlic and ginger.

- Cheese, ham and bacon all contain tyramine which increases our adrenaline levels, so pizza is out as a late-night snack too. Tyramine is found in raspberries, soy sauce and chocolate as well. Tyramine raises blood pressure and causes the release of the brain stimulant, noradrenaline.

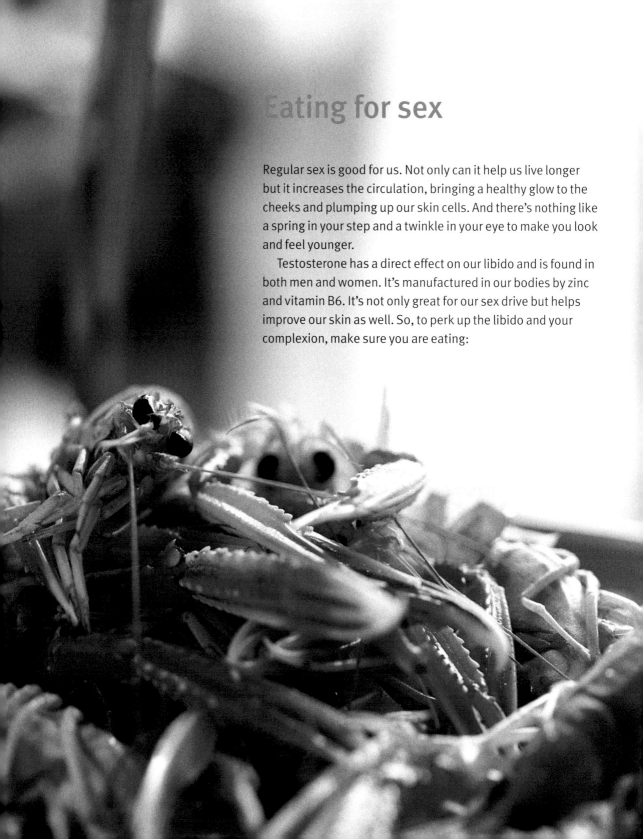

Eating for sex

Regular sex is good for us. Not only can it help us live longer but it increases the circulation, bringing a healthy glow to the cheeks and plumping up our skin cells. And there's nothing like a spring in your step and a twinkle in your eye to make you look and feel younger.

Testosterone has a direct effect on our libido and is found in both men and women. It's manufactured in our bodies by zinc and vitamin B6. It's not only great for our sex drive but helps improve our skin as well. So, to perk up the libido and your complexion, make sure you are eating:

···⟩ **Zinc-rich foods** – eggs, cheese, pumpkin and sesame seeds, shellfish, turkey, lentils, brown rice, wholewheat bread, peanut butter, fresh peas, watercress, figs and, appropriately, passion fruit. In particular, oysters are the richest source of zinc, so great for fertility, the libido and our skin.

···⟩ **Vitamin B6-rich foods** – potatoes, tuna, avocados, potatoes, bananas, chicken, chickpeas.

···⟩ **Vitamins A and E** – needed for the production of sex hormones (which drive the libido). They are found in oily fish, green leafy vegetables, liver, nuts and seeds.

···⟩ **Serotonin** – not only calms and relaxes but it does wonders for the libido as well (see page 254 for serotonin-rich foods).

···⟩ **Chromium** – believed to increase the sperm count in men and the sex drive for both men and women. Chromium-rich foods include asparagus, whole grains, nuts and seeds (see page 158 for more information on chromium).

···⟩ The sex organs need vitamin C and magnesium to function. Keep your levels topped up by eating citrus fruits, peppers, green leafy vegetables, mangoes, kiwi fruit, guava.

Avoid

···⟩ Drinking too much alcohol. While a glass or two can be relaxing, too much can be tiring, can reduce the level of testosterone and increase oestrogen levels (in both sexes) which lowers the sex drive.

···⟩ Eating too much. Not only is this fattening but it's difficult to perform well (or at all) after you've over-indulged.

DID YOU KNOW?
A study by Duke University, North Carolina, found that people who had more sex of higher quality generally lived longer than those who didn't. » You burn between 7 and 25 calories during orgasm (Masters & Johnson). » The smell of cinnamon buns has been shown to increase male sexual arousal. » Men can lose up to 3mg of zinc per ejaculation.

Eating for brain power

Your brain needs the right food to develop and remain active, just as your bones, muscles and organs require the right nutrients to grow and function properly. Researchers at the Institute of Brain Chemistry in London have shown that a baby's brain development in the womb is intimately linked with the amount of essential fatty acids their mother eats and in particular the amount of Omega-3 and DHA (docosahexaenoic acid) from oily fish. And this strong link continues throughout our lives with EFAs vital for healthy brain function (see page 112 for more information on EFAs).

The right nutrition not only affects the mechanical processes controlled by our brains, but also our mood. Scientists have now established links between behaviour and food including problems like Attention Deficit Hyperactivity Disorder (ADHD) in children, aggression, depression and even psychiatric problems like schizophrenia. As well as more serious problems, the wrong food can make us sluggish or forgetful; and what about that shakiness you get from drinking an extra cup of strong coffee or the extreme irritation that seems to come from nowhere when you've just binged on too much sugar?

DID YOU KNOW?
Foods rich in vitamin B can improve your memory. A study published by the Life Extension Foundation in the US found B vitamins helped in the production of actetylcholine, a neurotransmitter which controls brain speed. » Greek students burn rosemary when studying for exams to help remember the facts.

'There's rosemary, that's for remembrance.'
WILLIAM SHAKESPEARE, HAMLET

Top 10 brain boosters

1 Oily fish – they supply all the vital essential fatty acids your brain needs to stay healthy, as well as protein.

2 All fish, including shellfish – important both for the slow-release protein they contain and for minerals, including zinc, magnesium and chromium, found in shellfish such as oysters.

3 Nuts and seeds – also for protein but more importantly for the essential fatty acids and vitamins they supply. Nuts are an important source of boron – a trace element which, studies suggest, is vital for the transmission of electrical impulses in the brain.

4 Fruit – both fresh and dried supply energy and all-important vitamins and minerals, including antioxidants.

5 Bean and seed sprouts – not only alfalfa but also adzuki, garbanzo, lentil, mung, pea, peanut and a range of others. These are an excellent and delicious way to boost your brain power, supplying vitamins A, B, C and E, calcium, iron, magnesium, phosphorus, potassium, EFAs and protein.

6 Oats and other whole grains – your brain needs a steady supply of energy just like the rest of your body. Oats in particular help keep blood circulating.

7 Vegetables – the fibre, vitamins and minerals supply energy, and antioxidants.

8 Purple, red and blue fruits and vegetables – especially beetroot, blueberries, blackberries and pomegranates – are such a rich source of antioxidant flavonoids that they really help your heart, veins and arteries and increase the blood and oxygen flow to the brain.

9 Rosemary – Shakespeare and the ancient Romans can't be wrong. Rosemary works on the adrenal system. It stimulates the memory, improves concentration, can ease tension and anxiety, and soothe emotions. Include it in cooking, but also burn the essential oil to boost concentration. It's also great for digestion and cleansing our lungs.

10 Meat, eggs and dairy products – these are a good source of protein for slow-release energy, vitamins like D and minerals such as zinc. They are also an excellent source of essential amino acids (which the brain needs to function properly) and iron. Choose lean cuts of meat and semi-skimmed milk to reduce your intake of saturated fat.

Eating for eyesight

Along with the rest of the body, eyes show the signs of age. Aside from eye disease associated with ageing, eyes lose their brightness and can look red and watery. It's essential to have your eyes checked regularly by a qualified optician who will notice any changes in your vision as you age but also spot the first signs of disease at a point where it is still possible to treat and contain any eye damage.

However, there are nutritional choices you can make to keep your eyes as healthy as possible.

⇝ Antioxidants, including vitamins A, C and E may protect the lens against damage by free radicals.

⇝ Vitamin A is particularly good for eye health, so make sure your diet contains plenty of dark, leafy greens and orange and yellow-coloured fruits and vegetables which contain beta-carotene, an antioxidant-rich form of vitamin A.

⇝ Vitamin C and the antioxidant flavonoids found in dark red-purple berries, fruits and vegetables may be especially protecting for the lens.

⇝ Eye doctors recommend avoiding foods that cause rapid swings in blood sugar levels as these may increase your risk of developing glaucoma.

⇝ Herbs can be helpful when drunk as a tea or infusion. You can also use them as an external treatment as a compress or eye wash. Chamomile, fennel and eyebright are particularly good for fighting infection as well as soothing red eyes.

⇝ Ophthalmologists also stress the importance of a balanced, varied diet including Omega-3 fatty acids.

⇝ Supplements of zinc, melatonin, ginkgo biloba, bilberry and co-enzyme Q10 may also help eye health (see page 154).

Age-related macular degeneration

This is usually referred to as AMD and it is one of the most common degenerative eye diseases. The macular are the densely packed cells which allow us to see colour and fine detail and when they are damaged or begin to break down, central vision is impaired.

···› Researchers have found that the intake of antioxidant-rich food is very important, reducing the risk of AMD (and also cataracts).

···› Egg yolks are particularly effective as they contain lutein and zeaxanthin which are responsible for the yellow pigment. These are the only antioxidants that are transported specifically to the macular.

···› Lutein is also found in dark green vegetables such as broccoli and kale, but researchers calculate that lutein in eggs may be as much as 300 per cent more absorbable than that from vegetable sources.

DID YOU KNOW?
Rosemary may help to get rid of those dark circles and under-eye bags. Not only is rosemary an antioxidant, it also stimulates the circulation and helps to cleanse the liver which reduces puffiness and improves overall skin vitality. » Elderberries may help to strengthen vascular tissue in eyes and improve circulation.

DID YOU KNOW?
Studies show that supplementing the diet with vitamins C and E, beta carotene and zinc reduces the risk of developing AMD.

Eating for hormones

Eating for the menopause

The menopause isn't a disease. It's just something that happens at a certain time of life; like a first period, it's a rite of passage through womanhood. At this time, a woman's ovaries stop producing oestrogen. Some women sail through with hardly any symptoms; others experience hot flushes, a drop in energy levels, mood swings, joint pain and night sweats. One major effect can be an increasing dryness of the skin.

Whether you're taking HRT or not, a healthy diet can help you get through the menopause. It's a great boost for keeping your hormones on the straight and narrow which will make you feel a whole lot better. And if you feel good, you look good. Eating foods that are rich in hormone-balancing oestrogens, calcium and other healthy vitamins and minerals can reduce the unpleasant side-effects of the menopause.

DID YOU KNOW?

In Japan, menopausal symptoms are so rare there isn't a word for 'hot flushes'. » Oestrogen levels fall after the menopause, which means skin becomes thinner and more fragile and skin tone tends to become more uneven. » Hot flushes can affect around 70 per cent of menopausal women.

Foods to ease the menopause

--> Moisturize inside and out: eat lots of Omega-3 foods (sardines, salmon, mackerel, herring); use olive and flaxseed oils in cooking and in dressings; keep your vitamin E levels topped up (lots of avocados).

--> Cut down on coffee, alcohol and spicy foods, especially during hot weather. They encourage the blood vessels to dilate which means more sweating – not much fun if you're already prone to hot flushes.

--> Watch your blood sugar levels. Eat slow-release carbohydrates (whole grains, vegetables, beans, lentils) to keep your mood swings under control.

--> Nuts, seeds and oily fish are full of essential fatty acids that help ease joint pain.

--> Foods rich in fibre (whole grains, fruit, oats, beans, vegetables) help balance hormones.

--> Calcium levels need to be topped up as postmenopausal women are more vulnerable to osteoporosis. Eat canned sardines (with the bones), green leafy veg and low-fat dairy products.

--> Chickpeas, lentils, mung and aduki beans are full of phytoestrogens called isoflavones, which are great at reducing hot flushes and sweats.

--> Chamomile tea is a great body balancer. Either drink it as a tea or have a relaxing footbath with five drops of chamomile oil.

--> Using soya flour can reduce hot flushes by up to 40 per cent. A study at the University of California found that postmenopausal women who took a soya supplement twice a day had better verbal recall and were sharper thinkers than those taking a placebo. It's also good for your bones; the bone-building cells in women who drank soya milk were found to be more active than in those who didn't.

--> Tofu is made from the curds of soybean milk. Eating it regularly can help your cholesterol levels by 30 per cent. Amazingly, research is also showing that tofu can protect men against baldness. There's not much taste to it but it's great at picking up the flavours of food that it's cooked with.

--> Known to help boost the memory, sage can help reduce menopausal hot flushes, so use it when you're cooking. Put a couple of dried leaves in a cup, cover with boiling water and leave to infuse for an hour. When it's cool, drain. Then, take a tablespoon of the liquid each hour until the hot flushes stop.

--> Supplements such as dong quai, evening primrose oil, agnus castus and wild yam can help ease symptoms and improve skin quality.

Eating to ease periods

Ah, the swings and roundabouts of the menstrual cycle, where oestrogen and progesterone dosey-do with each other throughout the month. The natural rhythm of our monthly cycle is not just about fertility and reproduction; it helps our bodies maintain smooth skin, supple muscles and healthy bones – all of which are part of looking and feeling more youthful.

However, as many women will know, that monthly cycle has its downside. And it's hard to look (or feel) young and lovely when your stomach is cramping and you're holding onto more water than the Hoover Dam. What we eat can have a positive effect on the very negative symptoms of PMS. The more balanced your diet, the more oestrogen and progesterone you produce which is good. Women with lower levels of these hormones tend to suffer from PMS more than others.

PMS is an umbrella-term for a variety of symptoms:
⋯▸ food cravings
⋯▸ heavy periods
⋯▸ mood swings
⋯▸ water retention
⋯▸ weight gain
⋯▸ sore and swollen boobs

DID YOU KNOW?
Research shows that 70 per cent of young women regularly use painkillers to cope with the pain, and at least 50 per cent say it seriously disrupts their lives. ≫ There are more than 150 symptoms associated with PMS.

You often find that during the week before your period you will feel a bit tired and run down. Avoid the temptation to get a quick fix by grabbing a chocolate bar because the sugar surge and then sudden dip will make you feel even worse (and does nothing for the quality of your skin). Concentrate on eating foods that give a slow release of energy (see page 240). During your period, especially if your periods are heavy, you need to up your intake of iron-rich foods (such as chicken, sardines, egg yolks, dried figs, pulses such as chickpeas and kidney beans, spinach).

⋯⟩ A well-balanced diet, heavy on fish, fruit, vegetables, beans and pulses, and whole grains, but light on meat can minimize the effect of PMS.

⋯⟩ High levels of essential fatty acids can help minimize sore boobs and period pains, so opt for Omega-3 and -6 rich foods, such as fish.

⋯⟩ Evening primrose or borage oil are also good sources of essential fatty acids and are useful supplements at this time.

⋯⟩ Chasteberry (or vitex) is another supplement that keeps our hormones balanced. It stimulates the pituitary gland which increases production of a luteinizing hormone which, in turn, increases the production of progesterone in the second half of the menstrual cycle. It's also helpful in reducing period pains and the tender feeling in the breasts (NB Don't take if you are pregnant or on HRT).

⋯⟩ Organic meat and vegetables don't contain added pesticides and hormones which can affect our natural balance of oestrogen and progesterone.

⋯⟩ Minimize stress (see page 253 for a stress-busting food plan). Stress raises the levels of cortisol which competes with progesterone.

⋯⟩ If you suffer from PMS, make sure your diet is rich in B and C vitamins.

⋯⟩ Vitamin C is believed to strengthen uterine blood vessels so they are less likely to get damaged. This could reduce the length of bleeding and minimize heavy bleeding.

⋯⋗ Chromium and magnesium help to minimize sugar cravings (see pages 158–159 for foods rich in these minerals). A banana smoothie is a good idea, rather than a bar of chocolate.

⋯⋗ Avocados are full of vitamin B6 which helps to reduce PMS; eat regularly a week before your period.

⋯⋗ Keep drinking water. You need the fluid to flush salt out which is responsible for fluid retention. In other words, the more water you drink, the less likely you are to suffer from fluid retention. Increase your water intake to about 3 litres (5½ pints) the week before your period

⋯⋗ Potassium also helps to keep fluid levels down. Bananas and tomatoes are a good source, as are most fruits and vegetables.

Avoid

⋯⋗ Processed foods, ready meals, coffee, black tea, sugar.

⋯⋗ Salt, which can increase fluid retention. Use herbs and spices to flavour foods.

⋯⋗ Caffeine – it's a diuretic but, because it removes water so quickly, it leaves the salt in your body behind … which leads to fluid retention so you become locked in a vicious cycle. Caffeine also messes up the natural hormonal change and so can increase PMS symptoms.

⋯⋗ Too many animal fats.

DID YOU KNOW?
Chasteberry is from the 'chaste tree', so called because it was believed that the ripe fruit would lower the libido of women.

'Eat to live, and not live to eat.'

BENJAMIN FRANKLIN

The thyroid and thyroxine

The thyroid gland produces the hormone thyroxine. This controls most bodily functions, including skin and muscle repair, as well as helping to generate energy and burn fat. Selenium, zinc and iodine are essential nutrients for thyroid function.

If the thyroid is performing poorly and not producing enough thyroxine we burn food more slowly. If the opposite is true and the thyroid's gone into overdrive, food is burnt much faster; too fast to get the full benefit of the essential nutrients.

⋯⟩ Avoid eating broccoli, Brussels sprouts, cabbage, kale and cauliflower because they inhibit the absorption of iodine.
⋯⟩ Best sources of iodine: shellfish, seaweed, onions.
⋯⟩ Best sources of selenium: brewer's yeast, onions, nuts and seeds (especially brazil nuts), tuna.
⋯⟩ Best sources of zinc: oysters, sardines, pumpkin seeds, eggs, cheese.

DID YOU KNOW?
1 in 5 women suffer from some form of thyroid disease. It's difficult to spot because the symptoms (tiredness, anxiety) are often put down to normal, everyday stress.

Intolerances and allergies

Food allergies

These are reactions by the body to a particular food. The immune system kicks in immediately and starts producing antibodies to attack the protein to which you are allergic. Immediate symptoms can be itching, a rash, breathing difficulties, headaches, vomiting, body swelling and, in severe cases, collapse (anaphylactic shock). Allergies are usually present at birth. Food allergies are diagnosed by either a skin-prick or patch test or a RAST test (Radio Allergo Sorbent Test). If you are confirmed with a food allergy, the only safe treatment is to completely avoid that food.

Just eight foods cause over 90 per cent of all food allergies:

- Milk
- Fish
- Shellfish
- Gluten
- Peanuts
- Soya
- Tree nuts (eg brazil, walnuts, almonds)
- Eggs

Food intolerance

This doesn't trigger an allergic reaction but does cause the digestive system to react. Intolerances are not usually life-threatening. The most common is a lactose (milk sugar) intolerance, with up to 10 per cent of northern Europeans suffering from this. Symptoms can be wind, bloating, diarrhoea, abdominal pain, vomiting. A food intolerance can develop at any time but it can be managed and, in some cases, overcome by healthy eating. Some scientists believe an intolerance occurs if you eat too much of one thing. For example, a cereal breakfast, sandwich lunch and pasta supper means wheat at every meal.

DID YOU KNOW?
Some 'healthy' foods are actually bad for some people. There's often confusion, though, between a food allergy and a food intolerance.

Foods that cause common intolerances:

- Milk
- Eggs
- Wheat
- Soya

- Chocolate
- Caffeine
- Wine
- Some food additives

If you suspect you have a food intolerance, take your pulse, then eat the suspected food and take your pulse again. If it has increased by 10 beats per minute, you may be intolerant so seek medical advice.

Setting the balance

Having to avoid certain foods means that you can affect the 'healthy' balance of your diet. Avoiding milk and dairy products also means you miss out on a lot of key vitamins and minerals which can affect your general health and your skin condition.

Wheat allergy

You may not get enough B vitamins, iron, magnesium or potassium.
- Orange juice, fruits, leafy greens, pulses contain folate.
- Pulses and leafy green vegetables contain magnesium.
- Meat and fish contain iron and potassium.

Milk allergy/intolerance

You may not be getting enough calcium or phosphorus.
- Tofu, soya milk, canned salmon, spinach and broccoli contain calcium.
- Meat, fish, eggs and whole grains contain phosphorus.
- Vitamin D helps the body take in more calcium.

DID YOU KNOW?
1 in 5 people believe they are allergic to a food. In fact, less than 1 per cent of the adult population has a true food allergy; 20 per cent of the population has adverse reactions to food (British Dietetic Association). » Half of all adults in the UK who have asthma also have allergies (Mayo Clinic).

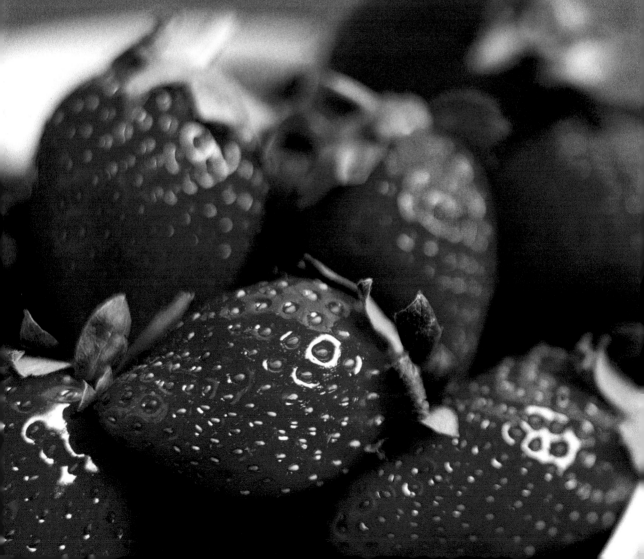

CHAPTER SIX

choosing youthful foods

If you've reached this point in the book, you should already have a fairly good idea of the types of foods you should be eating to remain healthy and hold back the signs of ageing. There is a clear message from dieticians and experts that it is vitally important to eat a balanced range of food with plenty of antioxidants to counter the ageing effects of free radicals.

To ensure our food delivers all the nutrients we need, it must be fresh and in optimum condition. There is no doubt that much of what's readily available just isn't very fresh. And with regular scare stories about everything from pesticide residues in vegetables, antibiotics in meat and chlorine in bagged salads through to the dangers of farmed salmon, it's hard to know what to choose to ensure what we're eating really is healthy and nutritious.

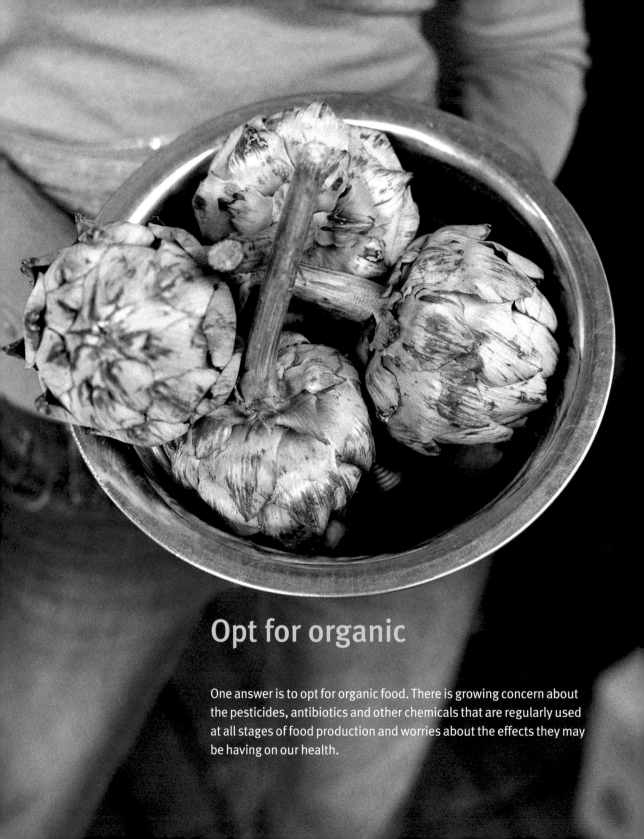

Opt for organic

One answer is to opt for organic food. There is growing concern about the pesticides, antibiotics and other chemicals that are regularly used at all stages of food production and worries about the effects they may be having on our health.

Chemicals in food – the facts

⋯⋗ 31,000 tonnes of chemicals are used on UK farmland each year.

⋯⋗ This figure includes 4.5 billion litres of pesticides.

⋯⋗ 350 different types of pesticide can be used legally in the UK.

⋯⋗ Many of the chemicals used were originally developed from chemical weapons and nerve gas during the Second World War.

⋯⋗ Experts estimate that roughly a quarter of our food is contaminated by pesticide residue.

⋯⋗ Almost 50 per cent of bread tested in 2003 showed significant traces of pesticide residues.

⋯⋗ Because many chemicals penetrate the plant's surface, simply washing fruit or vegetables doesn't always help.

⋯⋗ Chemicals can damage wildlife and spoil the natural balance of ecosystems and soil.

Why should we worry?

Pesticides have been linked with a number of age-related health problems including:

⋯⋗ A weakened immune system

⋯⋗ Weakened DNA and cell repair

⋯⋗ Accelerated gene loss

⋯⋗ A breakdown of the body's ability to detoxify itself

⋯⋗ Neurotoxicity, or age-associated brain damage

⋯⋗ Parkinson's disease

⋯⋗ Infertility

⋯⋗ Some cancers

Alongside all these are the fundamental ageing effects of free-radical damage, triggered by the chemicals in our bodies.

DID YOU KNOW?
The Maastricht Ageing Study in 2000 linked exposure to pesticides with a number of long-term side-effects. Farmers and gardeners were thought to be at particular risk.

LOSS OF NUTRIENTS
A 2002 research study in Canada found that over the last 50 years nutrient levels in non-organic potatoes had dropped dramatically. They had lost 100 per cent of their vitamin A, 57 per cent of their vitamin C and iron and 28 per cent of their calcium. The same pattern was found in a range of other vegetables and fruit. » A number of British studies also showed that vitamin and mineral contents had fallen markedly even when fresh produce was stored in supposedly ideal conditions.

Organic food is more nutritious

Organic food will always be fresher and therefore more nutritious. It also cuts down our consumption of toxins, including pesticides, antibiotics, artificial additives and GMOs (genetically modified organisms). Organic standards dictate that farmers must use good farming practice, with sustainable and environmentally friendly methods of producing food. Food labelled organic must comply with strict legal standards.

DID YOU KNOW?
Non-organic apples are often sprayed up to 16 times with a toxic cocktail of 36 different chemicals before they appear on shop shelves. They can also be kept 'asleep' for up to 12 months in sealed cold stores to preserve them. » The average non-organic lettuce can be sprayed up to 15 times with a variety of chemicals and pesticides. » The average non-organic fruit or vegetable will have been sprayed with pesticides, rinsed in chlorine, gassed or cold stored to slow deterioration.

Organic facts:
- Organic food is pesticide- and GM-free.
- Analysis shows organic products have higher nutrient levels with typically around 27 per cent more vitamin C, 29 per cent more magnesium and 21 per cent more iron as well as other vital vitamins, minerals and essential acids.
- Higher standards of animal welfare are guaranteed.
- Organic farming is better for the environment as the natural balance and fertility of soil is maintained.
- There is greater biodiversity. A Soil Association report in 2000 showed 40 per cent more birds, twice as many butterflies and five times as many arable plants.
- Energy consumption tends to be lower and energy efficiency higher so there are lower levels of harmful waste emissions, including between 40 and 60 per cent less carbon dioxide, the main global warming gas.
- By opting for organic, you'll not only be saving your own skin but helping the environment, too.

A WEIGHTY ISSUE
The lettuce you chose as the healthy, low-calorie option may not be doing you as much good as you think. One reason for using pesticides and chemicals in agriculture is to promote growth and plump up the product as quickly as possible. And the residues left behind can have a similar effect on you. Antibiotics and growth promoters used in animal farming are designed to do the same.

Going organic

If you can't afford to go wholly organic, choose organic versions of the foods you eat the most often. Another option is to replace the most chemically contaminated fruits and vegetables with organic.

Among the worst polluted fruits and vegetables are:

- Root vegetables, including carrots and potatoes
- Apples
- Apricots
- Grapes
- Peaches
- Cherries
- Pears
- Peppers
- Spinach
- Beans
- Broccoli

This is quite a shocking list, including many of the fruits and vegetables I'm most likely to eat because they are healthy, but it is important to keep a sense of perspective.

DID YOU KNOW?
Organic milk is better for you. A 2005 study by the Danish Institute of Agricultural Sciences found that organic milk was 50 per cent higher in vitamin E, 75 per cent higher in beta carotene, and a staggering 200–300 per cent higher in the antioxidants lutein and zeaxanthine than non-organic milk. It also confirmed earlier findings by a UK study that organic milk contains significantly higher levels of Omega-3.

My view

I personally don't think it's necessary to only buy organic food. For a start it's more costly, so for most people it is just not a practical option. I also still maintain that it's better to eat lots of fruit and vegetables rather than less because you cannot afford organic ones. I do, however, think it is worth investing in organic dairy products if nothing else. More importantly, as long as you eat a balanced diet incorporating lots of the super foods mentioned in this book, you will be well on your way to looking and feeling younger.

Antibiotics in meat

Antibiotics are regularly given to farm animals, including chickens, laying hens, beef and dairy cattle, pigs and fish. Obviously there's no question about their use to treat a sick animal but, in reality, antibiotics are more often used to promote speedy growth and to prevent infection.

The Compassion in World Farming Trust (CIWF) believes that antibiotic use in factory farming is largely to compensate for a lack of hygiene and poor farming practice where animals are kept in overcrowded, unhealthy conditions. The World Health Organisation voiced its concerns over the possible side-effects on human health, calling for a ban on their routine use as long ago as 1997. But despite this, the overall use of antibiotics in farming has gone up.

The implications for health are serious. Antibiotic residues remain in meat and meat products. Not only are people affected by the growth promoters remaining but there are increasing fears about the links between antibiotic use and the rise of superbugs – bacteria which have developed a resistance to commonly-used antibiotics.

Many of the antibiotics used for farm animals are very similar to those used to treat people. Bacteria are widely exposed to them on farms and develop a resistance. Scientists fear this is one of the reasons why many antibiotics previously used to treat human illnesses are no longer effective.

The CIWF believes resistant bacteria transfer from animals to people through:
⋯⟩ Meat
⋯⟩ Eggs
⋯⟩ Milk
⋯⟩ Vegetables or fruit grown in manure containing resistant bacteria
⋯⟩ Food preservatives

Seasonal sense

I still get really excited by the changing seasons – the first frost on spiders' webs in autumn, crisp winter days, pale green shoots in spring and long balmy summer evenings... OK, I know it's not all like that but you get the general idea. At the end of summer, however much you loved that new summer wardrobe back in May, aren't you impatient for change and to snuggle into that soft, new sweater or delicious suede boots?

So why don't we all feel the same way about food? Why do we carry on choosing the same meals whatever the season and weather? By eating with the seasons we will automatically be matching our body's needs with the food available at the right time. We can also guarantee that what we are eating is fresh, packed with nutrients and not damaged by long periods of storage or transport. And it's better for the environment.

I'm convinced this is the key to getting the most from food, and finding a guilt-free, more youthful you in the process. For a table showing when fruit and vegetables are in season, see pages 236–237.

'But doth not the appetite alter?
A man loves the meat in his
youth that he cannot endure
in his age.' WILLIAM SHAKESPEARE

Farmers' markets

There's no better or more fun way to shop for seasonal food than in a farmers' market. These used to be the preserve of the countryside, but now with so many opening in towns and cities, urbanites can benefit too.

On a typical weekend, my local farmers' market is buzzing. I never realized just how delicious freshly picked English apples could be. Now I can understand why there's such enthusiasm for them and I'm beginning to know my Worcesters from my Russets, Cox's from Crispins. And there's an enthusiasm about the place which makes food shopping a real pleasure. Much of the produce is organic but even when it isn't, it is always freshly picked and nearly always unsprayed. So you can find peppery watercress that was still growing first thing that morning and the last of the late strawberries that actually smell of strawberries.

As well as fresh vegetables and fruit, you will commonly find cheese (including goat, sheep and even buffalo varieties), fish, meat, preserves and freshly pressed juice. If something is unfamiliar, ask how to cook or prepare it – the growers and producers will usually know and be delighted to tell you.

Farmers' markets are a fun, interesting way to put you back in touch with nature, the seasons and what your body needs. For more information and a list of farmers' markets, visit the National Association of Farmers' Markets at www.farmersmarkets.net.

Shopping at your nearest farmers' market also makes sure the food you are eating is really fresh and local. It will have been grown nearby and so will be packed with nutrients and all the goodness it should contain. No time will have been wasted in transport or storage. That's better for you and also better for the environment.

Food miles

Although most supermarkets now stock a very comprehensive range of foods, much of the produce is from abroad and has flown very long distances. This clocks up 'food miles' which is the term scientists use to describe the environmental effects of the distances we transport our food.

Food mile facts:

- Only five of every 100 fruits bought in the UK will have been grown here.
- 76 per cent of supermarket organic fruit and vegetables comes from abroad.
- A single calorie of carrot flown in from South Africa uses 66 calories of fuel.
- The supermarket ingredients for a standard meal could have travelled over 38,000km (23,600 miles).
- Health problems associated with greater food mile distances include the spread of diseases and the loss of nutrients.
  (Source: Sustain – the alliance for better food and farming.)

Vegetable box schemes

Organic box schemes have seen business soar by 20 per cent in the last decade. They are now widely available throughout the country and offer a very efficient service. Many will also let you choose a selection rather than just having one box available.

They are based on the idea of selling fresh, seasonal produce which is locally grown without chemicals. The food produced won't have been stored or treated and should be full of nutrients and flavour. By buying through such a scheme, you will be supporting local growers, boosting your own nutrition and helping the environment.

See pages 236–237 for a guide to what's in season each month.

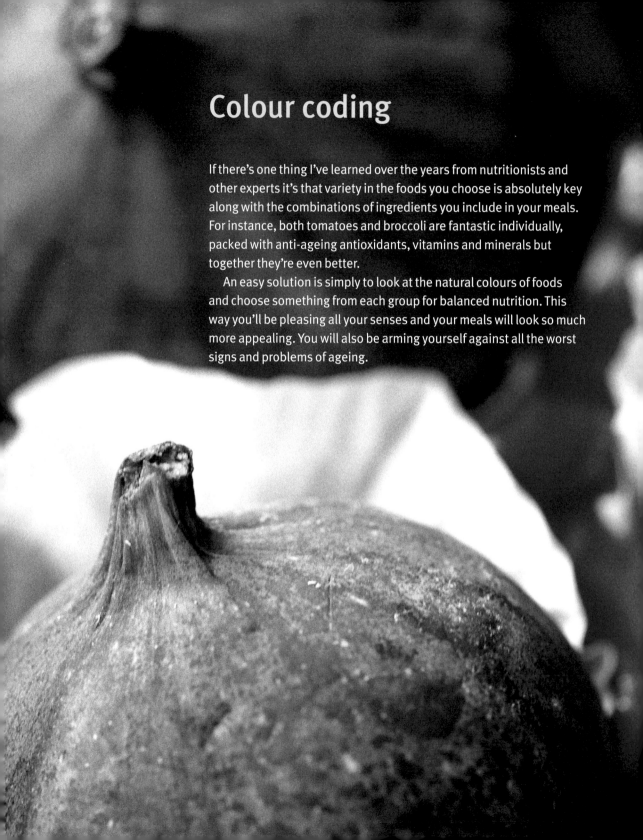

Colour coding

If there's one thing I've learned over the years from nutritionists and other experts it's that variety in the foods you choose is absolutely key along with the combinations of ingredients you include in your meals. For instance, both tomatoes and broccoli are fantastic individually, packed with anti-ageing antioxidants, vitamins and minerals but together they're even better.

An easy solution is simply to look at the natural colours of foods and choose something from each group for balanced nutrition. This way you'll be pleasing all your senses and your meals will look so much more appealing. You will also be arming yourself against all the worst signs and problems of ageing.

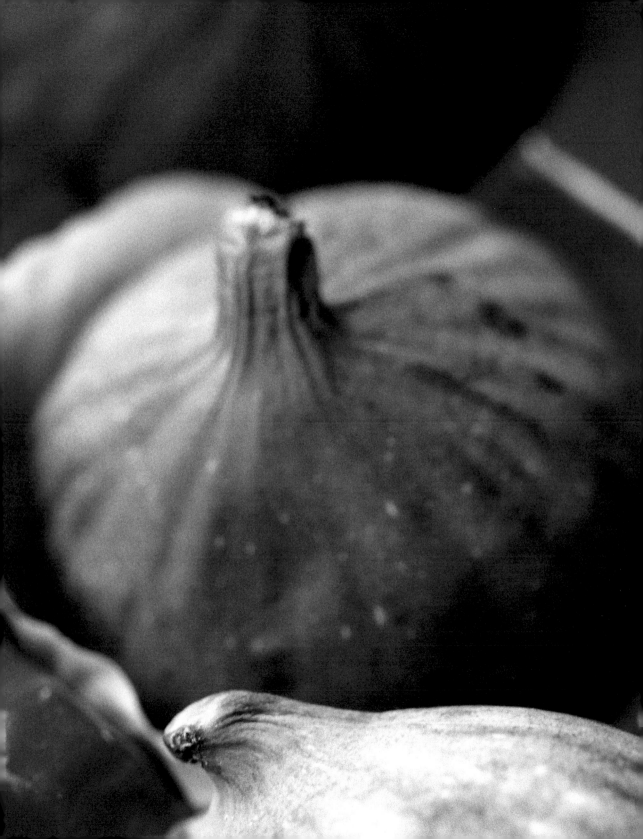

Red, yellow and orange

Fruits and vegetables in this group are powerful antioxidants containing high levels of vitamin C, carotenes and other nutrients.

⟶ They boost your body's defences against stress, pollution, chemicals, smoke and the sun.

⟶ They protect cells and cell membranes, including the skin.

⟶ They are anti-inflammatory, cut your risk of cancer and support your nervous system.

⟶ They contain high levels of vitamin C to protect against colds and flu.

These factors combine to make foods in this group fabulous weapons against the signs of ageing.

Good anti-ageing choices include:

⟶ Apricots
⟶ Bananas
⟶ Carrots
⟶ Ginger
⟶ Lemons
⟶ Oranges
⟶ Papayas
⟶ Pomegranates
⟶ Red peppers
⟶ Saffron
⟶ Strawberries
⟶ Tomatoes
⟶ Turmeric
⟶ Sweet potatoes

DID YOU KNOW?
Choosing red, yellow and orange for food, and for napkins and candles to decorate the table, will encourage your guests to eat well. These colours stimulate the appetite and nervous system.

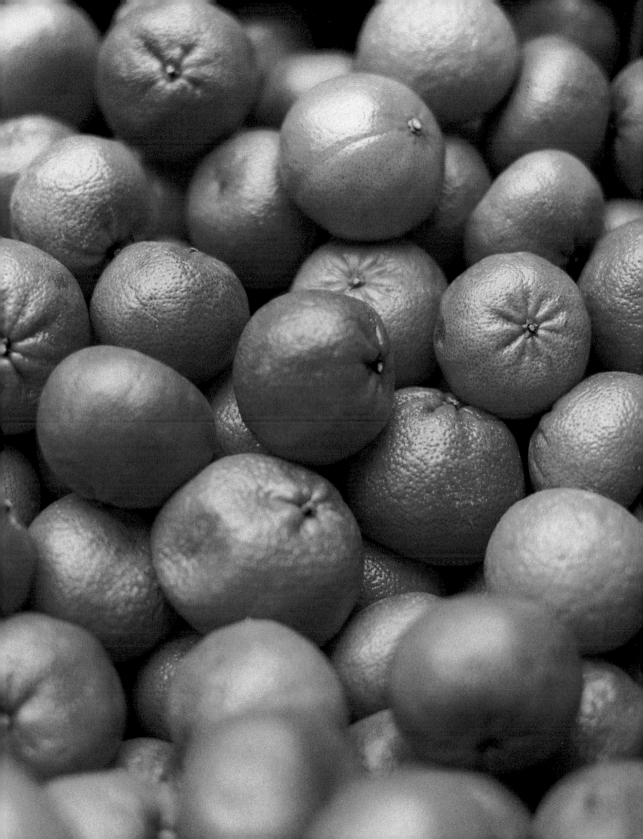

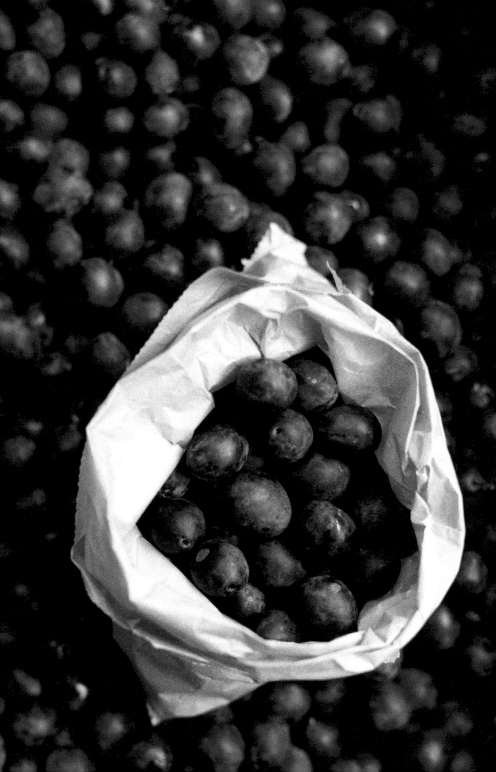

Deep red, purple and blue

The dense, deep colour is a sign of the high level of flavonoids this group of foods contain. Again, they are packed with vitamin C and are powerfully antioxidant and anti-inflammatory. The intense colour seems to match their strong, sweet flavours.

⋯⟩ These foods are good for your heart and cholesterol levels.

⋯⟩ They improve the function of your veins, arteries and circulation generally.

⋯⟩ They are natural antibiotics and useful for managing allergies.

⋯⟩ They protect body fluids.

⋯⟩ Many are listed among the top anti-wrinkle foods identified in the ORAC scale devised by Boston University (see page 36).

Top choices include:
⋯⟩ Aubergines
⋯⟩ Beetroot
⋯⟩ Blackberries
⋯⟩ Blackcurrants
⋯⟩ Blueberries
⋯⟩ Cherries
⋯⟩ Cranberries
⋯⟩ Figs
⋯⟩ Prunes
⋯⟩ Raspberries
⋯⟩ Red wine

DID YOU KNOW?
Flavonoids hold back an enzyme responsible for oestrogen dominance, which is an important factor in ageing and also some types of cancer.

DID YOU KNOW?
Use colourful spices instead of salt and pepper for great flavour and excellent anti-ageing properties. (See pages 146–148 for more information.)

Green

The green group of foods are antioxidant and detoxifying.

···∫ They are useful in the fight against wrinkles.

···∫ They contain high levels of sulphur which is good for your hair and skin. It is the sulphur which gives the distinctive smell when these foods are cooked.

···∫ These foods are also high in minerals like selenium, which boost your immune system and support your metabolism.

···∫ Selenium also helps the body absorb vitamin E and makes it more effective.

···∫ Green foods may help you lose weight as they regulate blood sugar levels and stop cravings for sugary, fatty foods.

Good greens include:

···∫ Asparagus
···∫ Broccoli
···∫ Brussels sprouts
···∫ Cabbage
···∫ Chives
···∫ Garlic
···∫ Kale
···∫ Kiwi fruit
···∫ Leeks
···∫ Onions
···∫ Spinach

DID YOU KNOW?
Pre-bagged salads may not be the healthiest choice. They are washed in a chlorine-based solution which means many of their nutrients are lost. As a response to public concern, some supermarkets now include unwashed bagged salads including organic wild rocket and watercress. These are a healthier option, preserving more of the antioxidant properties of the leaves.

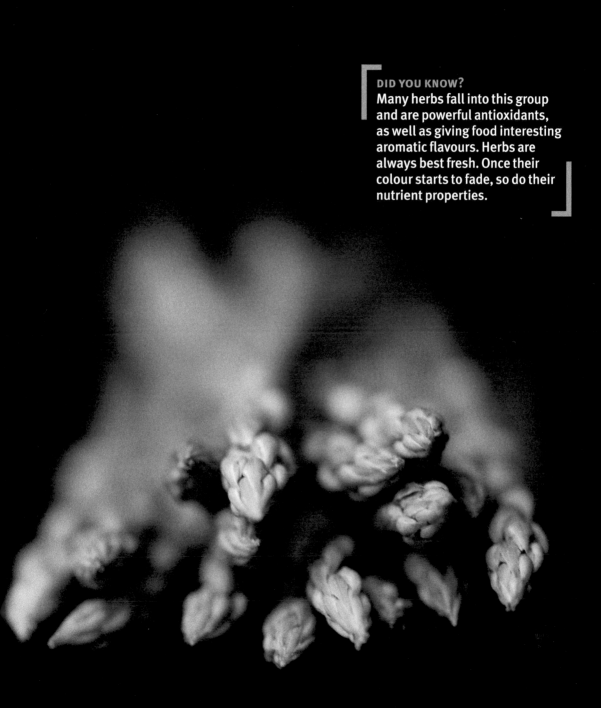

DID YOU KNOW?
Many herbs fall into this group
and are powerful antioxidants,
as well as giving food interesting
aromatic flavours. Herbs are
always best fresh. Once their
colour starts to fade, so do their
nutrient properties.

Brown

Foods in this group are full of fibre. They are generally satisfying, filling you up and helping to reduce your need for sugary foods. Avoid the processed white and go for the brown versions of staple carbohydrates like bread, pasta and rice instead. They will supply you with more complex slow-release sugars which are much better for your body, especially if you want to look younger for longer.

···→ The fibre helps your digestion and bowels, preventing your whole system becoming sluggish – a major factor in dull skin and cellulite.

···→ These foods are a good source of energy.

···→ They also help balance hormones.

···→ They contain vitamin E to protect cells and membranes.

···→ They are also rich in B vitamins, zinc, magnesium, chromium and other antioxidants.

···→ Many nuts and seeds in the group are brilliant sources of essential fatty acids and antioxidant minerals like selenium.

Best browns include:

···→ Almonds
···→ Beans
···→ Brazil nuts
···→ Brown basmati rice
···→ Brown mushrooms
···→ Chickpeas
···→ Couscous
···→ Lentils
···→ Sesame seeds
···→ Sunflower seeds
···→ Walnuts
···→ Whole grain bread

DID YOU KNOW?

The fibre and phytoestrogens in many brown foods actively work to lower harmful cholesterol levels and are powerful anti-cancer agents.

White and pale yellow

This group of foods are full of protein. They are also good sources of calcium, amino acids, essential fatty acids, vitamin A and other antioxidants which make them great anti-ageing foods. These are obviously all naturally white or light-coloured – they are not processed or bleached.

⇢ Important for strong bones, teeth and for maintaining muscle mass as we age.

⇢ The essential fatty acids and Omega-3 that many foods in this group contain are vital for maintaining supple, healthy skin and joints.

⇢ They are also essential for boosting your memory and brain power.

⇢ They help to balance mood swings and avoid depression.

Healthy white and pale foods include:

⇢ Chicken
⇢ Eggs
⇢ Fish
⇢ Macadamia oil
⇢ Milk
⇢ Olive oil
⇢ Sesame oil
⇢ Soya milk
⇢ Tofu
⇢ Turkey
⇢ Yogurt

DID YOU KNOW?
Macadamia oil has a mild, nutty flavour and can be used for dressings or cooking. It also contains four times as much vitamin E as olive oil.

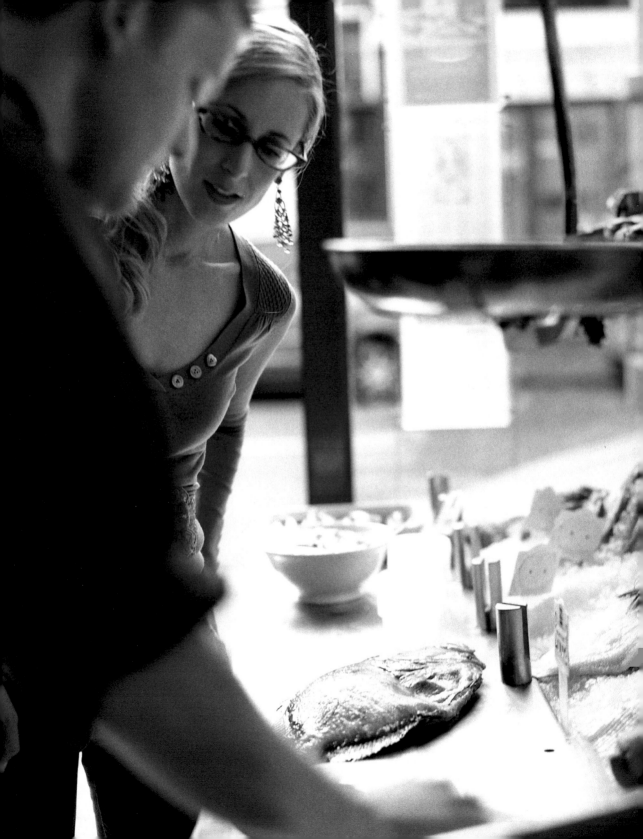

Go fishing

The message is clear. Fish is good for you. Fish consumption has been linked to a reduction of many ageing diseases. The fish oils found in oily fish (such as salmon, mackerel and tuna) are the best source of Omega-3 fatty acids which are vital for a healthy heart, brain development and good eyesight. They are also anti-inflammatory and reduce the risk of a range of ageing diseases. Alongside all this, they help to maintain smooth, wrinkle-free skin and supple joints. It's no surprise oily fish are so popular.

But it is increasingly important how you choose the fish you eat. There have been a number of scare stories about chemical pollutants and fish and it's hard to know the facts from the fiction. Salmon is a real super food – delicious and fantastic for you. But if you opt for farmed salmon, you could well be doing yourself more harm than good.

DID YOU KNOW?
Stocks of wild Atlantic salmon are overfished and it is now officially recognized as a threatened species. Pacific salmon have a shorter life span but are more prolific breeders and therefore not endangered.

Fishy facts

Here's everything you need to know about farmed fish, especially salmon. A survey by a US environmental working group found that farmed salmon were probably 'the most PCB and dioxin-contaminated protein source in the US food industry'.

PCBs and dioxins are chemical pollutants, waste products which come from a variety of sources including plastics and insecticide residues. Oily fish in particular absorb PCBs (polychlorinated biphenyls) and dioxins. These are toxins which are absorbed by fat. They cannot be broken down and so tend to build up to dangerous levels. They have been linked to a number of health problems for people. Farmed fish get most of their PCBs from their food – 'fish chow' – special pellets containing a mixture of ground-up fish, which may already be polluted, and oil. Many of the same factors which led to the BSE scare are at play here, because the fish chow increases the concentration of harmful substances in the fish.

PCBs and dioxins

⋯⋗ Thought to disrupt hormone function in humans.

⋯⋗ May trigger some forms of cancer.

⋯⋗ Affect the central nervous system.

⋯⋗ Pregnant women, anyone planning to become pregnant and children are recommended to eat no more than two portions of oily fish each week.

⋯⋗ It's thought safe for men to eat up to four portions a week.

DID YOU KNOW?
You can reduce levels of PCBs by removing the skin and any fat from the fish. Then steam, bake or grill which allows any fat (and with it any PCBs) to drain away, rather than frying where the PCBs are retained. Plenty of good Omega-3 oils will remain.

Farmed vs wild salmon

⋯⋗ Farmed salmon don't have the same opportunity to eat a variety of foods and algae that wild fish do.

⋯⋗ Colouring has to be added to farmed salmon food to give their flesh the characteristic pink colour. Without it they would be a dirty grey.

⋯⋗ Farmed salmon are kept in such confined, overcrowded pens that they need huge quantities of antibiotics and other drugs to keep them healthy.

⋯⋗ Antibiotic use has led to increases in antibiotic-resistant strains of bacteria which can cause disease in humans. They also make it more difficult to treat these diseases.

⋯⋗ Farmed salmon are also treated with pesticides to deal with the pests, including sea lice, they are prey to.

⋯⋗ A 2001 study in the UK revealed that farmed salmon contain up to 10 times the level of PCBs and dioxins found in wild salmon.

⋯⋗ They also contain higher levels of unhealthy saturated fats and lower levels of Omega-3 fatty acids compared to wild salmon.

⋯⋗ Farmed fish are frequently contaminated with other toxins including lead and heavy metals.

⋯⋗ Environmentally, farmed fish pose a threat to the wild species as they escape and cross-breed, weakening wild salmon stock.

The solution

⋯⋗ Choosing wild fish is the best way to limit the amount of PCBs and dioxins you are eating. Ocean caught fish are generally lower in toxins than those caught in lakes and rivers as oceans are obviously usually less polluted. The main exception to this is the Baltic which is one of the most polluted seas in the world. Worst of all are farmed varieties.

⋯⋗ Non-oily ocean fish such as cod and haddock have lean flesh which cannot store PCBs and dioxins, although their livers do store fat. Shellfish also retain lower levels of the toxins and supply some Omega-3 fatty acids.

The mercury debate

There has also been a great deal of concern over the amount of mercury which is found in all types of fish, not just oily types. Mercury is toxic to humans and can build up to cause poor concentration and vision, numbness and tremors. It's particularly serious for unborn babies because it can trigger brain and spinal cord damage.

I think the media play a big part in hyping up the mercury issue. The majority of us will never be affected by it so I really don't want this to put you off eating fish. The benefits you will get from increasing the amount of fish in your diet will far outweigh the chance of you experiencing mercury poisoning.

Worst affected fish:

⋯⃗ Albacore tuna
⋯⃗ Marlin
⋯⃗ Shark
⋯⃗ Swordfish

DID YOU KNOW?
Most of the tuna available in the UK is yellowfin or skipjack which does not have such high levels of mercury. Tinned tuna (with the exception of albacore) has lower levels than fresh.

How much oily fish should you eat?

The Food Standards Agency advises, 'Do not rely on fish from one source,' which applies to where it's caught as well as the variety of fish eaten. The government recommendation is for two portions of oily fish per week.

Good choices include ocean-caught:

⋯⃗ Anchovies
⋯⃗ Eels
⋯⃗ Herrings
⋯⃗ Mackerel
⋯⃗ Pilchards
⋯⃗ Sardines
⋯⃗ Trout
⋯⃗ Tuna
⋯⃗ Wild salmon and organic farmed salmon (see page 227)

Guilt-free fish and seafood

As well as health concerns over some fish, there are a number of ethical issues relating to how and where fish are caught. Various species face extinction from dwindling stocks due to over-fishing with drag-nets and poorly-managed waters where fish are caught out of season when they are spawning.

The Marine Conservation Society (MCS) publishes *The Good Fish Guide* which gives detailed information on everything to do with fish including fishing methods and management, marine life and lists of what to eat and what to avoid. Their website, fishonline.org, also gives easy access to information.

···᠈ As a general rule, the MCS recommends choosing line-caught fish as line fishing is far less damaging to ecosystems and other species, including dolphins.

···᠈ Wild ocean-caught fish tend to be less affected by pollution.

···᠈ Many species from North Atlantic and European waters are suffering from over-fishing. Pacific-caught fish are less affected.

···᠈ Cod stocks have been particularly decimated, so look out for line-caught fish from well-managed Norwegian or Icelandic waters.

···᠈ Fish have definite seasons. Find out what they are when selecting what to buy. (Look at the fishonline.org website.)

···᠈ Farmed fish doesn't have to be bad if you go for organically farmed fish or Freedom Food certified farms which ensure high environmental and welfare standards.

Readily available sustainable fish varieties include:
···᠈ Cape hake (MCS-certified)
···᠈ Dover sole
···᠈ Dublin Bay prawns
···᠈ King scallop (sustainably harvested)
···᠈ Lemon sole (not beam-trawl caught)
···᠈ Mackerel (line-caught or MCS-certified from Cornwall)
···᠈ Mussels (sustainably harvested)
···᠈ Oysters (farmed Native and Pacific)
···᠈ Pacific cod (line-caught)
···᠈ Pacific halibut (line-caught)
···᠈ Red mullet (not Mediterranean)
···᠈ Salmon (from the Pacific, MCS-certified from Alaska, farmed organic and Freedom Food certified only)
···᠈ Seabream
···᠈ Whiting
  (Source: Marine Conservation Society)

Ageing foods – what to avoid

Having looked at how to choose food and what to eat, it is also important to know what to avoid. So exactly what are the ageing disasters as far as food goes?

Salt

Too much salt is bad for your health. You've probably noticed government adverts setting out their guidelines that adults should eat no more than 6g of salt per day. 6g of salt is roughly equal to one teaspoon.

⋯⟩ Salt is the common name for sodium chloride and it is sodium that is most damaging to health.

⋯⟩ Around 26 million people in the UK eat more than 6g per day.

⋯⟩ An excess can causes high blood pressure and damage your heart, and increases your risk of a stroke.

⋯⟩ On food labels you may not be aware of just how much salt is actually present. Often it will be labelled as sodium. To find out how this relates to your daily intake of salt, you multiply the amount of sodium by 2.5.

⋯⟩ Get into the habit of checking labels and get to know what really is low salt.

⋯⟩ Watch out for salt in processed and packaged food – even cakes and biscuits. White bread, take-aways, ready-made meals, smoked cheeses and meats, instant soups, stock cubes, hard cheese, sausages and burgers all tend to have high levels of salt, along with more obvious salted snacks like crisps and roasted nuts.

⋯⟩ Herbs, spices, onions, garlic and lemon can all be used instead of salt in cooking to add flavour. Always taste food before you add salt – during cooking and at mealtimes.

⋯⟩ Many canned pulses and vegetables have salt added. Look for the ones which state 'no added salt' or drain and rinse before use.

IT'S NEVER TOO LATE . . .
Graham McGregor, Professor of Cardiovascular Health at St George's Hospital, London stresses that it's never too late to improve your health. People over 60 who cut their salt intake to 6g reduce their risk of heart attacks by 24 per cent and of strokes by 31 per cent in a few days.

Processed foods and sugars

····⫶ These tend to be full of refined carbohydrates which are all high on the glycaemic index and push up blood sugar and insulin levels, stressing and ageing the body.

····⫶ US researchers found that the waist measurements of people who ate a lot of refined carbohydrates were three times bigger than those with healthier diets. For more on the glycaemic index and the importance of balancing blood sugar levels, see pages 50 and 83–84.

····⫶ Processed foods also bump up our salt intake and tend to be low in vitamins, minerals and other nutrients including essential fatty acids. The extra sugars they contain deplete your stores of vitamins and minerals.

····⫶ Sugar is one of the most ageing foods. It has a negative effect on digestion and can cause irritable bowel syndrome, depression, migraines and lack of energy. Sugar also destroys collagen production so skin is more likely to wrinkle and sag and joints will stiffen.

····⫶ The amount of sugar in processed foods is not always obvious as it is often lumped in with the total carbohydrate content. A quick guide is how far up the ingredients list sugar comes.

····⫶ It's worth remembering that sugar can come in various guises including: sucrose, glucose, dextrose, maltose, fructose, invert sugar, as well as more obvious ingredients like maple syrup, golden syrup, treacle and honey. The recommended daily amount for women is no more than 7 teaspoons a day.

DID YOU KNOW?
Fruit and honey will provide you with a natural, healthier and more satisfying alternative to processed sugars.

DID YOU KNOW?
Many cereals are surprisingly high in salt. Some own-brands of cornflakes are 10 per cent saltier than the sea. ⟫ 80 per cent of most people's salt intake comes from processed and ready-made food.

Trans fats

I've already talked about how bad these fats are for you on page 82. They are impossible for the body to break down and have been implicated in a range of ageing health problems. They'll certainly add to your weight and have been linked with an increased risk of cancers. Watch out for them in processed cakes and biscuits, low-fat spreads, deep-fried foods and other processed snacks. Trans fatty acids, hydrogenated fat and hydrogenated vegetable oil are all other names for the same thing, and all are to be equally avoided.

Saturated fat

Too much saturated fat is associated with a number of age-related diseases including diabetes, heart disease, clogged arteries, strokes and a greater risk of cancers like breast, colon and stomach cancer. It is found in meat and dairy products. By choosing low-fat dairy options you will derive all the benefits without the damaging fat.

'All the things I really like to do are either immoral, illegal or fattening.' ALEXANDER WOOLLCOTT

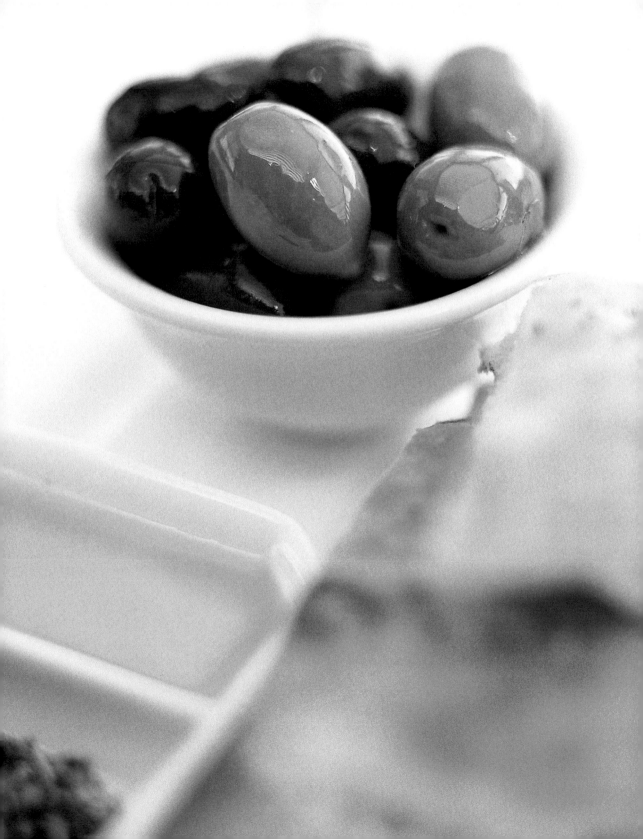

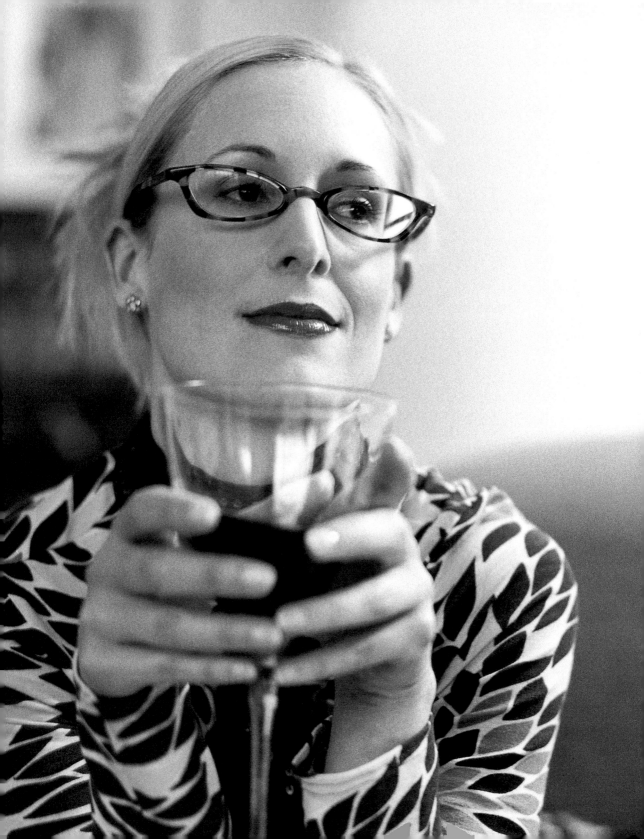

Alcohol

Yes, one or two glasses of wine are positively good for you. What I'm talking about here is drinking to excess. It's easy to spot a heavy drinker by the broken capillaries and ageing blotches.

Even at normal levels, alcohol dehydrates your body and skin. As it's a diuretic, it also robs your body of vital vitamins, minerals and other nutrients. It interferes with your circulation which shows in your skin as broken veins, wrinkles and a dull complexion.

It can also cause memory problems. Your brain cannot detoxify alcohol, so if you drink so much that your liver cannot cope with any more, the alcohol starts to dissolve the fatty acids in your brain cells.

On a positive note, in moderation a glass or two of wine can help you relax. Young red wines are also good sources of antioxidants. In particular, a flavonoid called resveratrol is a compound found mainly in red grape skins. It helps to control cholesterol levels and is thought to guard against heart and liver diseases as well as being an anti-cancer agent.

⋯⋗ If you know you will be drinking, make sure you also eat.

⋯⋗ Drink plenty of water to avoid the worst dehydrating effects and help prevent a hangover.

⋯⋗ Work on the basis of one glass of water to each glass of wine.

⋯⋗ Eating plenty of fruit and vegetables will supply you with antioxidants to counter the most ageing effects of the alcohol.

⋯⋗ Increasing your intake of vitamins C and B will help detoxify you.

⋯⋗ Milk thistle can also help support and detoxify your liver (see page 168).

Seasonal fruits, vegetables and nuts

FRUIT	Jan	Feb	Mar	Apr	May	Jun	Jul	Aug	Sep	Oct	Nov	Dec
Apples	×								×	×	×	×
Apricots					×	×	×	×				
Blackberries									×	×	×	
Blackcurrants						×	×	×	×	×		
Blueberries								×				
Cherries						×	×					
Elderberries								×	×			
Figs								×	×			
Grapes								×	×			
Peaches						×	×	×	×			
Pears							×	×				
Plums							×	×	×			
Pomegranates									×	×	×	×
Quinces										×	×	
Raspberries							×	×	×			
Redcurrants							×	×	×			
Rhubarb			×	×	×							
Strawberries					×	×	×	×				
VEGETABLES												
Asparagus					×	×						
Aubergines								×				
Beetroot						×	×	×	×			
Broad beans						×	×	×				
Broccoli		×	×	×		×	×	×				
Brussels sprouts	×											×
Cabbages	×	×										×
Carrots	×	×	×				×	×				×
Cauliflower									×			
Celeriac	×	×	×	×								×
Celery								×				×
Chicory								×				×

VEGETABLES	Jan	Feb	Mar	Apr	May	Jun	Jul	Aug	Sep	Oct	Nov	Dec
Courgettes							×	×				
Cucumbers							×	×				
Fennel								×				
French beans							×	×				
Garlic							×	×				
Globe artichokes								×				
Jerusalem artichokes	×	×										×
Kale	×	×	×	×								×
Leeks	×	×										×
Lettuces					×	×	×	×				
Mangetout						×	×	×				
Onions							×	×				
Parsnips	×	×	×	×								×
Peas						×	×	×				
Peppers								×				
Potatoes								×				
Radishes					×	×	×	×				
Rocket		×	×		×	×	×	×				
Runner beans							×	×				
Spinach	×	×			×	×	×	×				×
Swede	×											×
Sweetcorn								×				
Tomatoes						×	×	×				
Turnips	×	×	×									×
Watercress			×	×	×	×	×	×				
NUTS												
Almonds									×	×	×	
Hazelnuts							×	×				
Walnuts										×	×	

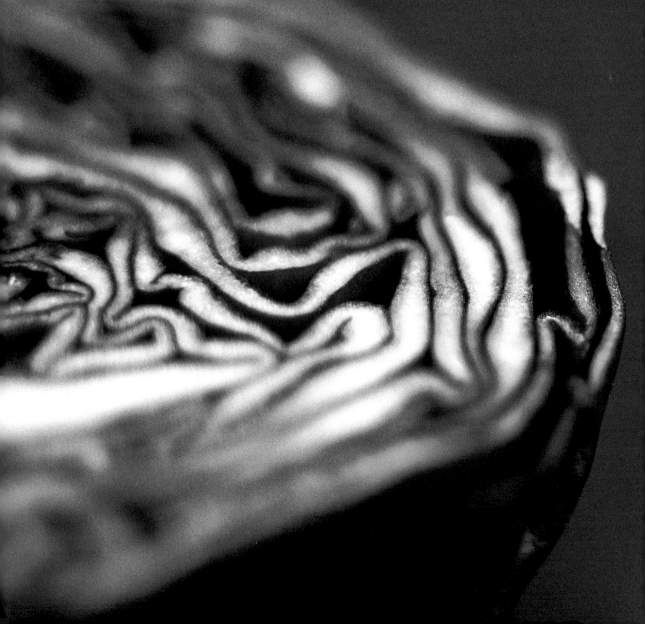

food plans

Breakfast is best

Skipping breakfast is an anti-ageing disaster. Research shows that people who regularly miss breakfast on average weigh an extra 3.5kg (8lb) and have higher harmful LDL cholesterol levels. Not only is it bad for your heart and your waistline, but you are also depriving your body of the fuel it needs for energy and to maintain vital body processes.

If you start the day well with a healthy satisfying breakfast, you are likely to feel more energetic, and less likely to crave unhealthy snacks and sugar. If you are in the habit of missing breakfast you will slow your metabolism, weaken your stomach and impair your digestive system.

Breakfast is the most important meal of the day and I never skip it, no matter how early I have to get up for filming.

DID YOU KNOW?
While you are sleeping your metabolic rate slows by 5 per cent. Eating breakfast literally breaks your fast, and revs up your metabolism so it goes back up to its normal rate.

Breakfast choices

My favourite choice is a bowl of muesli with plenty of fresh, seasonal fruit and natural, live yogurt. But there are other good options which will help to set you up for the day.

⋯⋗ The best breakfast combination is slow-release complex carbohydrates (like oats or whole grain bread) to boost concentration levels, protein such as milk, eggs or nuts which will maintain blood sugar levels for longer, healthy essential fats in the form of nuts, seeds or olive oil-based spreads, and fruit for added vitamins.

⋯⋗ Oats are a particularly healthy choice as they are full of soluble fibre, which is not only good for your bowels but helps keep cholesterol levels low and regulate hormones.

⋯⋗ Other good complex carbohydrates are oatmeal, whole grain or rye bread.

⋯⋗ Avoid eating the same thing every day. If you vary your food, you will make sure you are eating a wide range of nutrients and really supplying your body with what it needs.

⋯⋗ Whole grain cereal with dried fruits and nuts will supply a range of nutrients including antioxidants and essential fatty acids.

⋯⋗ Try poached eggs on whole grain or rye toast. Both these breads contain more complex, slow-release carbohydrates which will keep your energy levels steady for longer. Eggs are an excellent source of protein, vitamins and iron.

⋯⋗ If you really hanker for a cooked English breakfast, grill the bacon, tomatoes and mushrooms instead of frying and poach the egg.

⋯⋗ Another healthy and delicious traditional breakfast is kippers, or smoked haddock, and a poached egg.

⋯⋗ Or what about smoked salmon and scrambled eggs to boost your intake of Omega-3s, iron, vitamins and protein.

⋯⋗ Skip sugary cereals. They won't sustain you for very long, and will quickly be converted into glucose which prompts insulin production and can encourage the body to lay down fat.

···⟩ Don't ditch dairy – dairy foods sometimes get a bad press but unless you are allergic, they are an excellent source of calcium and if you opt for semi-skimmed milk or low-fat yogurt you will not be bumping up your intake of saturated fats.

···⟩ Some dieticians recommend soya milk but as certain cancers, including breast cancer, are affected by oestrogen, the plant oestrogens contained in soya may not make this a healthier option. If you want to avoid dairy, almond, oat or goats' milk may be better choices.

···⟩ Always make sure you drink something. Ideally first thing in the morning, get into the habit of drinking hot water and lemon to flush out toxins and kick-start your digestion. Then with your breakfast, try antioxidant-rich green, white or black tea. I never drink coffee but the milk most people add to it can be a useful source of calcium.

···⟩ It is better to eat a whole fruit rather than drink fruit juice at breakfast-time. Recent research from the Monell Chemical Senses Center in the US showed drinks like fruit juice and smoothies which are high in fructose suppress appetite-regulating chemicals in our bodies.

···⟩ Choosing a fruit rather than juice means you know it is fresh and unprocessed with a higher vitamin content. You'll also be gaining useful fibre and as the fruit takes longer to eat, your body will find it more satisfying and you'll be consuming fewer calories.

OAT FACTS
Oats are an excellent source of fibre and can reduce harmful LDL cholesterol levels. ⟩⟩ They are calming to the nervous system and can reduce sugar, caffeine and even nicotine cravings. ⟩⟩ Oats give you energy and help concentration. ⟩⟩ Oats can even help beat hangovers. ⟩⟩ They are also high in vitamin B6 which balances the testosterone-oestrogen ratio to improve libido and so boost your sex life.

Breakfast is best recipes

As well as the recipes that follow, try these breakfast suggestions:
- Energizing muesli and variations
- Oatmeal muffins
- Healthy eggs Florentine
- Vegetable omelette
- Kedgeree
- Whole wheat pancakes with fruit
- Mixed seed, nut and fruit bread
- Hazelnut and raisin bread

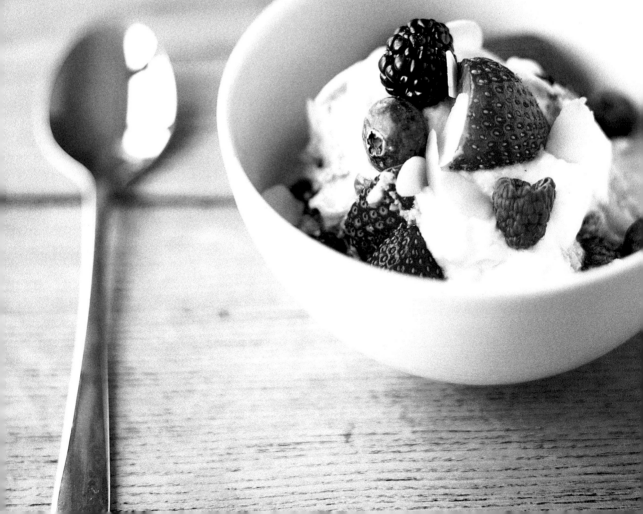

Muesli with toasted nuts, seeds, fresh fruit and yogurt

Whole grain cereal flakes are the perfect breakfast food as they provide you with a sustained release of energy. Oats are particularly rich in soluble fibre, B vitamins, iron, magnesium and zinc. Soaking the cereal flakes in milk overnight makes them softer and easier to eat. In this recipe, they are mixed with heart-healthy flax seeds (which provide a near-perfect balance of Omega-3 and Omega-6 fatty acids) and vitamin C-packed summer berries.

SERVES 2

85g (3oz) mixture of oats, millet flakes and rye flakes
300ml (10fl oz) skimmed or semi-skimmed milk
30g (2 tbsp) sultanas
30g (2 tbsp) toasted flaked almonds, chopped hazelnuts
    or cashews
30g (2 tbsp) flaxseeds (ground)
225g (8oz) berry fruits, eg blueberries, blackberries,
    strawberries, raspberries
1 apple, peeled and grated
15ml (1 tbsp) honey (optional)
15–30ml (1–2 tbsp) natural bio-yogurt

1 In a large bowl, mix together the cereal flakes, milk, sultanas, nuts and ground flax seeds. Cover and leave for at least 2 hours, preferably overnight, in the fridge.
2 To serve, stir in the berry fruits, grated apple and honey (if using). Spoon into cereal bowls, then top with the natural bio-yogurt just before serving.

Porridge with raisins and cinnamon

Starting the day with a bowl of porridge gives you a fantastic energy boost. I like to add chopped fresh fruit – try sliced banana, blueberries, strawberries, clementine segments or any other fruit that takes your fancy. Oats are rich in soluble fibre – excellent for improving digestion and lowering blood cholesterol – as well as iron, B vitamins, vitamin E and zinc. They provide slow-release energy to sustain your energy through the morning. The dried and fresh fruit provide extra fibre and vitamins.

SERVES 2

85g (3oz) rolled porridge oats
125ml (4fl oz) skimmed milk
125ml (4fl oz) water
30g (2 tbsp) raisins, sultanas, dried apricots or dates
5ml (1 tsp) cinnamon
30g (2 tbsp) chopped toasted almonds
125g (4oz) fresh fruit (see above)

1 Mix the oats, milk and water in a saucepan. Bring to the boil and cook for approximately 5 minutes, stirring frequently.
2 Stir in the raisins, cinnamon and almonds. Spoon into bowls, and top with fresh fruit.

Winter warmers and immune boosters

Winter is a wonderful season – a time of crisp walks through woods full of falling leaves, wrapping yourself up in warm jumpers, snuggling up by a roaring fire, waking up to a world dusted with frost and lit by wintery sun. I may have grown up with the South-African sun, but I appreciate and enjoy winter here as well. It's also the season when the nights draw in and colds and flu abound, so if you want to stay bright and fighting fit throughout the winter you need to eat the right foods and give your immune system a boost.

Winter wisdom

···⟩ Keep drinking fluids. We tend to drink less at this time of the year but it is important to keep your fluid levels up. Not only does this plump up your skin but it helps your immune system too. If you're dehydrated, your immune system is compromised. Central heating also saps your skin of moisture so it's important to continue to drink as much water as possible.

···⟩ We are all guilty of eating fewer fruits and vegetables in the winter. Juicing is a great way to get more into your daily diet. Try a combination of parsley (vitamins A and C), lime juice (vitamin C) and carrots (full of carotenes) for a great winter health booster.

···⟩ Try to use seasonal food. It tastes better and hasn't flown halfway round the world. Root vegetables are much more nutritious at this time of the year because all their energy reserves are in their roots to avoid the cold.

···⟩ Roast some winter vegetables to concentrate their natural flavours, sprinkle with chopped garlic and drizzle with olive oil (full of Omega-9 fatty acids).

···⟩ It's really important to eat foods rich in vitamin D at this time. We usually get most of this vitamin from the sun but winter sun just isn't strong enough. Our vitamin D reserves halve every six weeks so during the winter months so it can be difficult to keep those levels topped up. You can get vitamin D from oily fish (such as mackerel), eggs and cheese.

···⟩ It's natural to want to eat more in the winter. Our ancestors needed the extra calories to build fat to keep out the cold, but thanks to central heating, we don't need to do this anymore. So don't overload the plate; go for lean protein which will fill you up without piling on the calories.

Mood enhancers

There's always a danger that we can feel a bit low and gloomy in the winter months. You get up in the dark, go to work and come home in the dark. Where did all the sunshine go? Banish the winter blues by choosing the right foods.

⋯⟶ Avoid blood sugar surges which can adversely affect your mood even more.

⋯⟶ Eat protein-rich foods (like salmon, turkey, chicken, lentils) or complex carbohydrates (such as brown rice or wholemeal bread) which release blood sugar slowly.

⋯⟶ Keep a handful of sunflower seeds nearby. Full of essential vitamins and minerals, they also contain magnesium which can help fight depression.

⋯⟶ Bananas are full of tryptophan which the brain uses to make the 'feel good' hormone, serotonin. Whizz up a banana with some other fruit, such as apples or pears, and some plain live yogurt to start the day with a spring in your step.

⋯⟶ Game (such as pheasant or guinea fowl) is rich in B vitamins, iron and tryptophan to help keep you looking on the bright side of life.

⋯⟶ All types of rice contain tyrosine, an amino acid which is used to make adrenalin and noradrenalin which, in turn, help us to get motivated. Leafy vegetables and milk are also good sources of tyrosine.

⋯⟶ For a winter-warming treat, draw the curtains, light the fire and make yourself a smoothie. Blend a banana, some milk and plain yogurt together. Simmer in a pan, whisk and pour into a mug. Sprinkle some cinnamon and cocoa powder on top. Cinnamon is full of chemicals that are good for your heart and your digestion and act as a pick-me-up. Who needs hot chocolate when you've got this?

DID YOU KNOW?
By the time we reach 70, we will have spent the equivalent of three years suffering the effects of over 200 colds.

Weather watch

Your skin is the first line of defence against the elements. And the skin on our face is the thinnest on the body so needs extra protection. At this time of the year, you have to give your skin all the help it can get. Antioxidants will help strengthen your defences.

···❧ Vitamin A strengthens our skin inside and out so it's an important weapon against germs. Foods rich in vitamin A include carrots, sweet potatoes, pumpkin, eggs, papaya, yellow fruits, fish liver oil.

···❧ Oily fish and roasted vegetables will keep your Omega-3 and -6 levels topped up – vital for keeping your skin looking hydrated and healthy.

···❧ Brazil nuts are a staple of the Christmas festivities. They're also a good source of Omega-6 fatty acids, an excellent source of protein and fibre and contain selenium which boosts the immune system.

···❧ Supplements such as starflower or evening primrose oil will keep your skin, hair and nails looking great. Scientists have found that taking evening primrose oil capsules every day has the same anti-ageing effect as expensive face cream (*International Journal of Cosmetic Science*).

···❧ Don't forget to protect your skin at this time of the year; use a moisturizer or foundation with an SPF.

···❧ Resist the temptation to turn up the central heating. It can suck the moisture out of your skin so easily and increase the danger of inflammation. Put on an extra layer and cuddle up to someone instead.

···❧ Keep positive. If you get stressed out, so does your skin.

···❧ A brisk walk gets the circulation going and gives you a healthy, pink, sexy glow.

···❧ Make sure you get enough beauty sleep; skin heals itself and regenerates at night.

Immune boosters

Central heating and air conditioning systems may keep the temperature at a comfortable level but they play havoc with our bodies. They dry up our mucus membranes which are a major defence against colds and germs.

Keep drinking fluids to hydrate your system; the body needs water to produce a steady stream of mucus to flush the germs out.

A pinch of cayenne pepper on your food helps reduce congestion.

Boost your probiotic intake – eat live yogurt or take multivitamins which contain probiotics. This enhances the immune system by increasing the release of defence cells that protect against viruses and bacteria.

Viruses hate vitamin C and can't thrive if there's any around. So keep your vitamin C levels topped up throughout the winter.

That apple a day just won't go away. Research shows that people who regularly eat apples are less likely to get colds and respiratory problem thanks to the high levels of vitamin C.

Apples are also a great aid to digestion. They contain malic acid which the body uses to break down food so nutrients can be absorbed more easily. Make some apple sauce to go with a roast dinner.

Apple skin contains up to five times more antioxidants than the flesh and two-thirds of the total fibre.

If you can't get hold of apples, try oranges, blackcurrants, blueberries and kiwi fruits.

Juice up some fresh oranges for a great fresh drink, full of vitamin C.

Frozen berries, such as blue-, black- and raspberries, are still full of antioxidants. Make a mental note to freeze them when they're around in the summer so you can still enjoy their goodness in the winter months.

Cranberries are one fruit that ripen much later in the year. Full of beta carotene and vitamin C, they are a great addition to your diet.

⋯⋗ Stewing some apples and pears (or other winter fruits) together with some lemon juice, spices and/or vanilla pods makes a great winter-warming compote that's full of vitamin C. If you haven't got fresh fruit, use dried instead (figs, prunes, raisins, apricots).

⋯⋗ Zinc keeps colds and flu at bay and, if you've already succumbed to a cold, can speed up your recovery if you increase the dose.

⋯⋗ Zinc is found in oysters, lean red meat, poultry, nuts and seeds, dairy products, shellfish, oats, rye and pumpkin seeds.

⋯⋗ If you're worried about colds, take a couple of zinc lozenges. NB Large doses of zinc can actually depress your immune system so don't go overboard.

DID YOU KNOW?
The world record for eating the most oysters in 10 minutes is 36 dozen. I don't recommend it!

Winter warmer recipes

As well as the following recipes for salmon and lamb kebabs, try these suggestions:

⋯⋗ **Kedgeree:** great for a hearty breakfast (fish: Omega oils; rice: tyrosine for mood; eggs: iron and vitamins; curry powder: boosts circulation).

⋯⋗ **Mackerel pâté:** good source of Omega oils and vitamin D.

⋯⋗ **Winter soups and stews:** for protein to fill you up and not pile on the pounds, such as chicken soup (Jewish penicillin) which boosts the immune system and protects our respiratory system; sweet potato soup (beta carotenes, vitamin C, antioxidants).

⋯⋗ **Pumpkin risotto:** pumpkin flesh is full of beta carotene and vitamin C (protects against infection); rice contains tyrosine to help us feel motivated. You could switch rice for pearl barley which has the same amount of calories but is higher in fibre than risotto rice and has a lower GI.

⋯⋗ **Curry:** chilli is an antioxidant and boosts circulation. Ginger contains vitamin C and acts as an antibiotic. Onions – protect against cold and flu; garlic – antiviral, antibiotic. Use tomato-based sauce (lycopene) and leave out ghee and cream. Curcumin (the spice that gives the yellow colour) is believed to activate an enzyme that protects the brain against oxidation – a major factor in ageing.

Other winter-warming foods to include in your daily diet

···› Garlic (boosts cell renewal and is antiviral, antifungal and an antibiotic).

···› Onions (high in sulphur which supports the immune system and detoxes the liver).

···› Green tea – protects against colds thanks to the bacteria-fighting chemical L-theanine.

···› Fish and lean meat (contain polysaccharides which are responsible for producing the immune-system cells).

···› Mushrooms also contain polysaccharides which boost the body's defences against infection.

···› Choose green leafy veg like kale, which is a very strong antioxidant vegetable and full of nutrients, or broccoli, packed with minerals, antioxidants, vitamins C and E, folate and iron.

···› Pelargonium is the new kid on the block as far as herbal remedies are concerned. Trials have shown that it can shorten the symptoms of bronchitis and tonsillitis by two days.

···› Echinacea, that old favourite of herbal remedies, helps build up resistance to colds and flu and boosts the immune system. Don't take it all through the winter; use it on a weekly basis, now and again to top up your immune system.

···› Freshly grated ginger in some hot water helps to flush out toxins, perk up your skin, stimulate your circulation and protect the immune system. And if you've already succumbed to a cold or virus, ginger is warming, comforting and eases sore throats and upset tummies. It contains anti-inflammatories called gingerols which reduce muscular aches and pains.

···› Red wine – research shows that if you drink red wine *moderately* (no more than a few glasses a week) you have a 40 per cent lower risk of getting a cold than those who don't imbibe.

Roasted winter vegetables with oat-crusted salmon

The lightly toasted oat crust makes the fish lovely and crispy on the outside while adding extra flavour and nutrients. Salmon is a concentrated source of Omega-3 fatty acids, which help reduce the risk of heart attacks and stroke, as well as benefiting the skin, reducing the appearance of wrinkles and also helping to control blood pressure.

SERVES 2

2 carrots, peeled and halved
1 parsnip, peeled and cut into quarters
1 medium red onion, peeled and cut into wedges
1 medium leek, sliced into 2.5cm (1 in) pieces
1/2 small butternut squash, peeled and thickly sliced
1 garlic clove, peeled and crushed
A few sprigs of fresh or dried rosemary
A little low-sodium salt and freshly ground black pepper
15–30ml (1–2 tbsp) olive oil
300g (10 oz) salmon fillet, skinned
30g (2 tbsp) porridge oats
15ml (1 tbsp) sesame seeds
Lemon wedges to serve

1 Pre-heat the oven to 200°C/400°F/Gas mark 6.
2 Prepare the vegetables and place in a large roasting tin. Scatter over the crushed garlic, rosemary, low-sodium salt and black pepper. Drizzle over the oil and turn the vegetables gently so they are coated in a little oil. Roast in the oven for 30–40 minutes until the vegetables are tender.
3 Meanwhile, cut the salmon in half. On a plate mix together the porridge oats and sesame seeds with a little low-sodium salt and black pepper. Dip each salmon portion in the oat mixture and press all over so that the oats coat the fish evenly.
4 Brush a non-stick frying pan or griddle with a little olive oil (or use an oil spray), heat then add the salmon. Cook over a moderate heat for 3 minutes on each side, covering with a lid. The salmon should be light brown and crispy on the outside.
5 Divide the roasted vegetables between two plates, place a salmon fillet on top and serve with the lemon wedges.

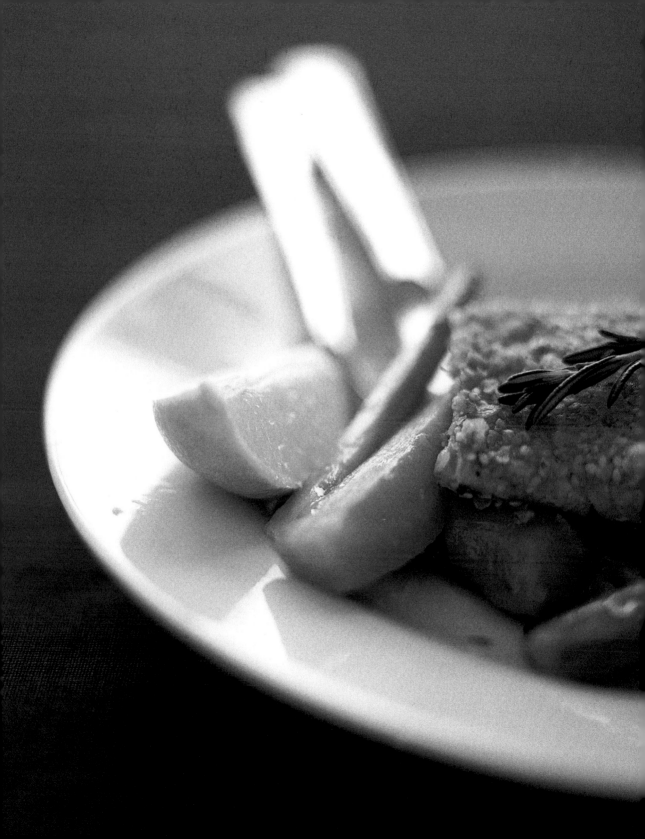

Lamb kebabs with caper dip

Lamb is an excellent source of easily absorbed iron, as well as zinc, protein and B vitamins. Choose lean steaks and trim off any visible fat – this reduces the fat content to around 9g per 100g.

MAKES 2 KEBABS
225g (8oz) lean lamb leg steaks
1 red onion, peeled and cut into wedges
25g (1oz) butter
1 sprig fresh rosemary

For the caper dip:
30ml (2 tbsp) capers, drained and rinsed
3 pickled gherkins, chopped
15ml (1 tbsp) wholegrain mustard
15ml (1 tbsp) white wine vinegar
15ml (1 tbsp) fresh mint, chopped
15ml (1 tbsp) fresh parsley, chopped
30ml (2 tbsp) mayonnaise

1 Cut the lamb leg steaks into 2.5cm (1in) cubes and thread onto skewers with the red onion wedges.
2 Melt the butter in a pan over a gentle heat and stir in the fresh rosemary leaves. Brush over the skewers and cook under a preheated grill for 12–15 minutes, turning occasionally.
3 Meanwhile make the caper dip: in a bowl mix together the capers, pickled gherkins, mustard, white wine vinegar, herbs and mayonnaise.
4 Serve the kebabs with the caper dip on a bed of healthy brown rice, and a large mixed leaf salad.

Stress buster

Stress is a part of our lives. It's nature's way of helping us cope with emergencies. But like so much in life, too much of anything can be harmful. Long-term stress means high blood pressure, tense muscles and poor digestion – hardly the ideal conditions for looking and feeling younger.

When we become stressed, we go into the 'fight or flight' mode and our bodies are flooded with adrenalin and the stress hormone, cortisol. Over a long time, this has a devastating effect on our bodies in general and our skin in particular. Skin sensitivity is increased, anti-inflammatories are released, blood sugar shoots up, our immune system comes under attack and our body starts to lay down excess fat reserves. Our stomach produces more acid which can inflame the stomach lining and limit our absorption of nutrients. Stress can also shorten the time it takes food to pass through our digestive system; so once again, we get fewer nutrients.

Cortisol is one hormone that we produce more of as we age. Many scientists call it the ageing hormone. What we eat and how we feel are inextricably linked. There are many ways to combat stress – eating is one of them.

If you are under a great deal of stress:

⋯⋗ Eat at least six small meals a day. When we feel anxious we produce adrenalin; this can cause blood sugar levels to drop dramatically so eating little and often will prevent this.

⋯⋗ Eat foods rich in vitamin C to protect your immune system which can come under attack when we're feeling emotional and overwhelmed. Include foods like red peppers, broccoli, kiwi fruit, watercress, blueberries, citrus fruit and melon in your diet.

⋯⋗ Vitamins B1 and C are especially good at keeping us calm and less anxious. The body can't store either vitamin in great amounts so they both need topping up regularly. Vitamin C is found in fruits, juices, leafy green vegetables, tomatoes, melons and potatoes; while foods such as rice bran, whole grains, peanuts, green and yellow vegetables, fruit and milk contain vitamin B1 (or thiamine).

> **DID YOU KNOW?**
> **Stress is the number one reason people take time off work.**

·····> Avoid following high-protein, low-carb diets because they increase mental activity. Not great if you're already feeling stressed. You want to wind down, not speed up.

·····> Eat 'good mood' foods (such as chicken or turkey; or complex carbohydrates like jacket potatoes, brown rice, pasta or beans) that are rich in tryptophan. Tryptophan encourages the production of serotonin in the brain. It's a mood enhancer, controls our eating patterns and acts as a natural sedative. If our serotonin levels are low, our bodies don't perform at their best.

·····> Other good sources of serotonin are walnuts, figs, avocados, bananas, pineapple, dates, papaya, aubergines.

·····> Treat yourself to *small* amounts of good-quality dark chocolate. Yes, it contains some caffeine but it also has theobromine, a chemical which stimulates endorphins (the feel-good hormones) in the brain.

·····> Calcium can help lift a feeling of depression; it does this by neutralizing lactic acid which is produced after physical activity or mental stress. Good sources of calcium are milk and dairy products, sesame and sunflower seeds, green vegetables, walnuts.

·····> Feeling anxious can be a sign of a nutrient deficiency; in particular, a deficiency of magnesium and zinc and the essential amino acid tryptophan. Make sure your diet includes plenty of nuts, whole grains, beetroot, fish, tofu, garlic, peppers, chickpeas, pumpkin seeds and cottage cheese.

·····> Take St John's wort, a natural mood enhancer, because it boosts our natural levels of serotonin.

·····> Siberian ginseng reduces anxiety and lemon balm acts as an antidepressant and sedative.

Eating throughout the day

Eating regular meals will keep your blood sugar levels on an even keel and stop you snacking throughout the day.

Breakfast

Breakfast is the key to feeling and looking good. Studies have shown that people who regularly eat breakfast were less depressed, less emotionally distressed and had lower stress levels than those who didn't. Scientists believe breakfast helps build a nutritional shield to protect against the negative effects of stress on the body.

···> Start the day with warm water and juice of half a lemon. This balances acidity caused by stress.

···> Muesli contains serotonin-boosting whole grains, nuts, seeds and dried fruit. Serve with natural yogurt and some fresh fruit to give yourself a dose of stress-busting nutrients that include zinc, vitamin C, B vitamins and magnesium. Essential fats in nuts and seeds help strengthen cell membranes and improve the moisture barrier property of the skin. Top with prunes so it's good for skin *and* your stress levels.

···> Porridge is full of slow-releasing carbohydrates that give you energy and help concentration. It's calming to the nervous system, can reduce sugar, caffeine and nicotine cravings and provide energy all morning. Instead of giving quick burst of glucose into the bloodstream (like most wheat-based cereals), porridge gives a steady trickle which is perfect for maintaining your concentration. Make with skimmed milk so it's low in fat but still a good source of calcium. Add a handful of dried fruit and have glass of orange juice to bump up your daily intake of fruit by two portions.

···> Add a spoonful of Manuka honey to your porridge if you like it sweetened; it has fewer calories than sugar. It can also help calm your nerves and has antibiotic properties.

···> Alternatively, start the day with an egg, a slice of wholegrain toast, a banana and six walnuts. You'll feel full for longer and won't experience the roller-coaster ride of blood sugar crashes and highs.

···> Take a multivitamin to make sure you are getting all the nutrients you need.

Mid-morning

···≀ Peppermint tea can boost brain power, relieve headaches and clarify thoughts. Its powerful menthol component helps relax muscle tension or stomach cramps from stress.

···≀ Four cups of tea (green, white, herbal) a day can reduce the risk of a heart attack by 11 per cent without over-stimulating you.

···≀ Avoid fatty foods; they make you feel sluggish during the morning. If you feel like this you're more likely to reach for stimulants like caffeine and chocolate to perk you up but that only gives you a quick rush, followed by an equally fast drop – and you're back where you started.

···≀ Eat an orange if you're getting wound up. Vitamin C helps combat anxiety and lowers stress hormones. One orange provides your recommended daily intake of vitamin C (a great antioxidant) and is a perfect mid-morning snack.

Lunch

···≀ Eat something for lunch. And, ideally, eat it away from your desk to give yourself some quality 'you' time.

···≀ Getting some fresh air and a change of scenery will help you feel better, allow you to enjoy what you're eating and make you more productive in the afternoon.

···≀ Fresh soup contains an incredible amount of nutrients and energy. With a warm liquid base, nutrients are carried round the body in the most efficient manner. Go for rich, hearty veggie soups.

···≀ Whole grain pastas with lots of vegetables are a good choice – the complex carbohydrates combine with the vegetables to release serotonin. It also provides long-sustaining energy for you to draw on throughout the day.

Mid-afternoon snack

- ⸱⸱⤳ If you need to nibble on something, snack on a small handful of almonds – a good source of essential fatty acids and also full of magnesium (low levels of magnesium can lead to tension, anxiety and irritability).

- ⸱⸱⤳ Magnesium is nature's tranquillizer. It works best with calcium, another mineral found in almonds.

Dinner

- ⸱⸱⤳ Avoid foods containing the amino acid tyramine (such as bacon, cheese, ham, red wine, avocados, raspberries, soy sauce) because they can keep you awake.

- ⸱⸱⤳ Instead, opt for foods like lettuce (which contains a natural sedative called lactucarium; Cos lettuce is ideal) or try turkey, tuna, bananas, figs or yogurt which contain sleep-promoting trytophan.

- ⸱⸱⤳ Increasing your vitamin B6 intake (low-fat milk, lean meat) will also help fight insomnia because our bodies need it to produce serotonin.

- ⸱⸱⤳ Make your freezer your best friend. When you prepare meals, make double the amount and freeze half. That way, you have nutritious, tasty meals ready in an instant. No more worrying about what to eat and whether it will be healthy or not. Soups, casseroles and stews are easy to freeze.

'Eat nutritionally, not emotionally.'

JORGE CRUISE, AMERICAN NUTRITIONIST

Throughout the day

···⟩ Avoid caffeine. Coffee drinkers have up to a third more stress hormones in their system than non-coffee drinkers, which means they are more prone to stress. High stress levels increase our blood sugar levels; if that sugar isn't used up it gets stored as excess fat. If you really can't do without that caffeine hit, drink no more than a couple of cups a day and then switch to herbal teas.

···⟩ Avoid alcohol or cut your consumption right back. It is a depressant which can increase mood swings.

···⟩ Avoid eating a lot of alkali-producing food, such as curry powder, black pepper and ginger which are believed to raise anxiety levels.

···⟩ Switch from white to brown. Whole grains are rich in thiamine (vitamin B1) without which we get moody and irritable. Getting cross means more frowning and that is very ageing!

In addition

···⟩ 20 minutes gentle exercise three times a week is a great way to beat stress. When you exercise, your brain releases powerful chemicals that give your mood a real boost. Endorphins, the body's natural pain reliever, are released whenever you exercise and will stay with you for the next eight hours. Slow breathing also helps release endorphins.

···⟩ Draw up a 'de-stress' list: ten things that make you feel happy and relaxed. If you feel under pressure, pick one thing from the list, a memory or a feeling, to help you feel calmer and less stressed. An image of walking by water always does it for me.

···⟩ Use all your senses: the smell of vanilla in drinks or foods can apparently help people deal better with stress.

···⟩ Take a relaxing bath with essential oils (lavender, ylang ylang) before you go to bed. Sprinkle lavender or jasmine essential oils on your pillow for a good night's sleep.

···⟩ You are not indispensable. Learn to say 'no' and delegate more. Make time for yourself. Take pleasure in the smallest things – a refreshing herbal tea in a favourite cup and saucer; a posy of flowers on your desk...

Stress-busting recipes

As well as the recipes that follow, try these stress-busting food ideas:
- Turkey salad
- Spicy chicken sandwich
- Avocado and prawns
- Brown rice salad/risotto

Butternut squash and sweet potato soup

This soup makes a great lunch when it's cold outside. It's really warming and tasty, perfect served with a slice of crusty wholewheat or rye bread. Butternut squash and sweet potatoes are both rich in beta-carotene, a powerful antioxidant that helps protect skin against UV light damage, wrinkling and premature ageing. Butternut is also a useful source of vitamin C, which is needed for making collagen, and sweet potatoes are rich in vitamin E, which is vital for healthy skin.

SERVES 2
1 small onion, peeled and chopped
1/2 medium butternut squash, peeled and cut into chunks
250g (9oz) sweet potatoes, peeled and chopped
1 garlic clove, peeled and crushed
5ml (1 tsp) grated fresh ginger
Pinch of freshly grated nutmeg (optional)
500ml (16fl oz) vegetable stock
15ml (1 tbsp) Omega-3-rich oil or extra-virgin olive oil
A little low-sodium salt and freshly ground black pepper
A small handful of chopped fresh coriander (or parsley)

1 Place the vegetables, garlic, grated ginger, nutmeg (if using) and vegetable stock in a large saucepan. Bring to the boil, lower the heat, cover and simmer for about 20 minutes until the vegetables are tender.
2 Remove from the heat and liquidize with the oil until smooth using a blender or food processor. Return to the saucepan to heat through.
3 Season the soup with low-sodium salt and freshly ground black pepper. Ladle into bowls and scatter over the chopped coriander.

Roasted peppers with rocket, couscous and almonds

One portion of this dish gives you your entire daily requirement for vitamin C. Red and yellow peppers are super-rich in vitamin C, as well as beta-cryptoxanthin and beta carotene, all powerful antioxidants that help defend against free radical damage and promote healthy skin, as well as helping combat the effects of stress, and protect the body from heart disease and cancer. The almonds in this dish provide extra protein and calcium.

SERVES 2

1 red and 1 yellow pepper
45ml (3 tbsp) extra-virgin olive oil
1 small onion, peeled and chopped
1 garlic clove, peeled and crushed
125g (4oz) couscous
Large pinch ground cinnamon
25g (1oz) toasted flaked almonds
A little low-sodium salt and freshly ground black pepper
50g (1 bag) ready-washed rocket

1 Pre-heat the oven to 190°C/375°F/Gas mark 5.
2 Cut the peppers in half lengthways, keeping the stalk attached, and remove the seeds. Brush the outsides with a little of the olive oil, then place them, skin-side down, in a roasting tin, packing quite tightly so they don't roll over.
3 Put the couscous into a large bowl and pour over 200ml (7fl oz) boiling water. Cover and leave for 10 minutes. Stir the cinnamon into the couscous and fluff up with a fork. Add the remaining olive oil, toasted almonds and seasoning. Mix well, and then spoon the mixture into the pepper halves.
4 Cover the roasting tin tightly with foil and bake for 1 hour until the peppers are tender. Take out of the oven and divide between two plates, then scatter over the rocket.

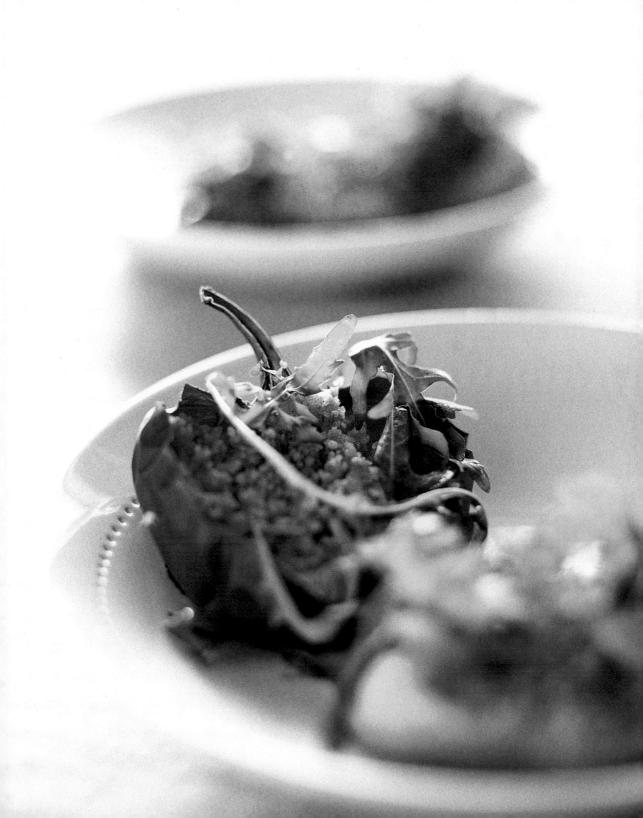

Cocktails and canapés

The actress Sandra Bullock once claimed that she used haemorrhoid cream to tighten up her skin and get rid of wrinkles. While I'm not disputing her claim, it's just not... well, very girly and fun. I've got a much better idea for banishing wrinkles and bringing a gorgeous glow to your cheeks.

Throw an anti-ageing cocktail party for all your friends. Get together and have a great time. Having fun, raising your energy levels and letting a love of life shine through does wonders for your skin and your friendships. Forget the haemorrhoid cream. At this party you get to eat your wrinkles away, pamper yourselves and have a fun night together all at the same time.

DID YOU KNOW?
Scientists at UCLA in California found that when women spent time with their women friends they released more of the hormone oxytocin which combats stress. >> Research from Harvard Medical School found that the more close friends and family we have, the better we age.

'Don't eat too many almonds; they add weight to the breasts.'
COLETTE, FRENCH AUTHOR

Canapés

If you don't want to bother with formal meals and sitting down at the table, go for canapés and provide a dazzling array of healthy – and tasty – finger food.

Here are some fab food suggestions:
⋯⟩ Grilled asparagus, drizzled with olive oil. Olive oil is full of Omega-9, which is good for skin inside and out. Extra-virgin olive oil contains strong antioxidants that combat the oxidizing effect of sun on skin.

⋯⟩ Quails' eggs – hard boil and serve with a twist of low-fat cream cheese on top. Eggs contain protein, vitamins B, A and D and sulphur which are all good for hair, nails and skin.

⋯⟩ King prawns, marinated in lemon juice, garlic and olive oil and threaded onto a skewer. Grill for a few minutes on each side until cooked. A good source of zinc and essential fatty acids.

⋯⟩ Mini salmon fishcakes make great canapés: full of iodine, protein, calcium, vitamin D and Omega-3s – great for preventing inflammation and creating glowing skin.

⋯⟩ Walnuts and almonds, served in bowls for easy nibbling, have anti-inflammatory properties to keep skin smooth and pimple-free.

⋯⟩ Hummus – contains chickpeas and tahini to provide energy and calcium.

⋯⟩ Pop some grapes in the freezer and serve cold.

⋯⟩ Peppers, carrots, tomatoes can be chopped up as crudités for the dips. They're full of antioxidants and vitamin C to combat free radicals. Red and dark orange peppers contain loads of vitamins A and E and bioflavonoids which help skin heal from within.

⋯⟩ Popcorn – also contains serotonin to help keep everyone in the party spirit.

⋯⟩ For a sweet tooth and dessert, serve chocolate-covered prunes and strawberries – tip the fruit in melted dark chocolate (chocolate contains serotonin to help the party go with a swing; it also contains magnesium and large quantities of flavonoids – good for the circulation which improves the complexion). Make sure chocolate contains at least 70 per cent cocoa solids. Prunes have extremely high levels of antioxidants. Strawberries contain ellagic acid which has been found to minimize the damage caused by pollution and smoke.

⋯⟩ Cut up lots of colourful, tasty fruit into bite-sized pieces and serve on cocktail sticks.

Cocktails

A glass or two of wine a day can be good for you. Serve a glass of Rioja or Cabernet Sauvignon to your guests at the party. Red wine contains powerful antioxidants (flavonoids) but have only a glass or two. Any more is harmful. Or make your own anti-ageing cocktails – see page 269 for some ideas.

Alternatively, for the drivers, non-drinkers and for the rest of the evening, you can provide anti-ageing drinks with a twist. For example:

⋯⋗ Elderflower spritzer (cordial plus fizzy water) – not quite the same as champagne, but delicious!

⋯⋗ English Rose (75ml cranberry juice, 30ml lychee juice, 20ml rose-petal syrup) – full of vitamin C and antioxidants so great for the skin.

⋯⋗ Orange and cranberry juice – the jewel-like colours of this drink are bright and vibrant. It looks and tastes zingy.

⋯⋗ Smoothies – blueberry and mango for a really heavy antioxidant punch.

⋯⋗ Mix orange juice, raspberries, strawberries, chopped-up watermelon and kiwi fruit and add a splash of apple juice for a powerful vitamin C fruit punch. Raspberries contain sulphur which is used to manufacture the connective tissues found in skin, hair and nails so helps to keep you looking young and is a component of insulin which helps regulate blood sugar (too much blood sugar destroys collagen); watermelon contains the antioxidants vitamin C and carotenoids; kiwi fruit is bursting with vitamin C.

'33 is the age at which the health benefits of moderate drinking begin.' THE LANCET

···> Alternatively, swap the raspberries, strawberries, watermelon and kiwi fruit for pineapple juice and ginger ale. Add the ginger ale just before you're ready to serve. Inflammation has an ageing effect on skin, but the pineapple contains bromelain which reduces inflammation, and ginger is a great stimulant so ideal for adding some fizz to the party.

···> If your party is in the winter, mix up a non-alcoholic mulled orange juice. Put some orange juice in a pan, add a cinnamon stick and a few cloves and simmer gently for 15 minutes. Remove the cinnamon and cloves before serving. Winter can be a time of colds and flu – not great for the party spirit or visions of youthful loveliness so we need to keep our vitamin C levels topped up. Oranges are full of vitamin C and will help boost your daily quota of iron. Cinnamon stimulates the efficiency of insulin so your body doesn't have to produce too much; great for good-looking skin because too much insulin has a damaging and ageing effect.

···> Try a prune 'Skin Smoothie': combine orange juice, 150g (5oz) strawberries, sliced banana, pitted prunes and some sliced peaches in a blender and mix until smooth. Prunes have the highest ORAC score which means they are stuffed full of anti-ageing antioxidants. The ellagic acid in the strawberries minimizes the damage caused by pollution and smoke, plus they're great at cleansing the system and keeping our skin looking glowing and healthy.

Cocktail and canapé recipes

As well as the recipes that follow, try
these suggestions:
⋯⋗ Tapenade
⋯⋗ Hummus
⋯⋗ Falafel

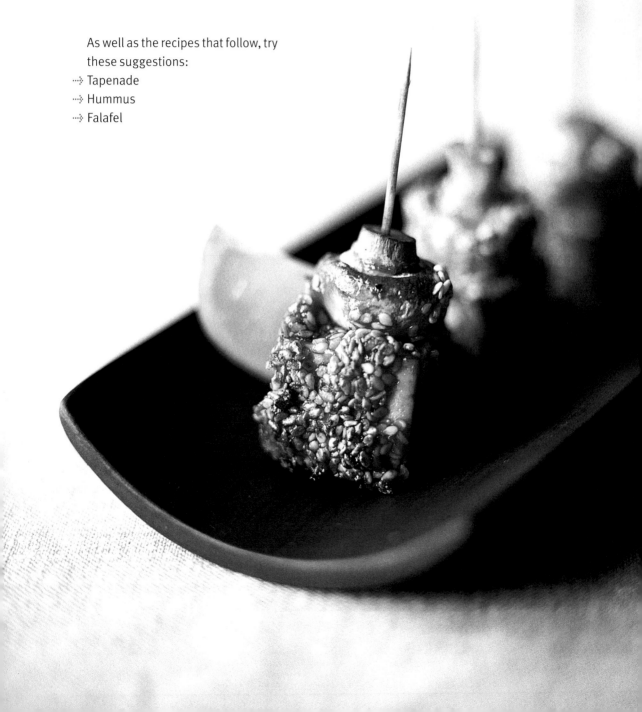

Tofu, mushroom and sesame brochettes with Szechwan sauce

Tofu is a great low fat protein source. It is also rich in bone-strengthening calcium and contains isoflavones, which help protect against heart disease, certain cancers and menopausal symptoms. In this recipe they are coated in sesame seeds, which are packed with calcium, iron and zinc.

SERVES 2

For the Szechwan sauce:
30ml (2 tbsp) soy sauce
15ml (1 tbsp) lime juice
20ml (4 tsp) sesame oil
10ml (2 tsp) rice wine vinegar
10ml (2 tsp) clear honey
10ml (2 tsp) sweet chilli sauce
1 garlic clove, peeled and chopped

8 cocktail sticks
125g (4oz) firm tofu, drained and cut into 8 bite-sized cubes
8 button mushrooms
30–45ml (2–3 tbsp) sesame seeds
Small lime or lemon wedges

1 Pre-heat the grill and line the grill rack with tin-foil.
2 First make the Szechwan sauce. Place all the ingredients for the sauce in a screw-top jar and shake well to mix.
3 Transfer the sauce into a shallow bowl and put the sesame seeds on a plate. Spear one tofu cube and one mushroom with a cocktail stick and dip them into the sauce. Roll in the sesame seeds until well-coated.
4 Arrange on the lined grill rack and grill the brochettes for 5 minutes, or until slightly browned. Turn frequently during cooking to avoid burning. Arrange on a serving plate and garnish with lime or lemon wedges.

Mini salmon fishcakes

All fish is rich in protein and important minerals. Salmon, in particular, is rich in the essential Omega-3 fatty acids, vital for controlling blood pressure, balancing hormones and promoting healthy skin. In this recipe, the fishcakes are coated in wholemeal breadcrumbs, which provide extra fibre, iron and B vitamins. Make your own, by whizzing wholemeal bread in a food processor, then spread the crumbs on a baking sheet and toast in the oven at 375°C/190°C/Gas mark 5 for 5 minutes.

MAKES 8 SMALL FISHCAKES

450g (1lb) potatoes, peeled
450g (1lb) salmon fillet, skinned
60g (2oz) butter
60ml (4 tbsp) milk
15ml (1 tbsp) fresh parsley, chopped

Grated zest of 1 lemon
A little low-sodium salt and freshly ground black pepper
1 egg, beaten
125g (4oz) oven-toasted wholemeal breadcrumbs
Rapeseed or olive oil for frying

1 Cut the potatoes into quarters and boil for 15 minutes until soft. Drain.
2 Meanwhile, poach the fish in water for 10 minutes. Drain and flake the fish, carefully removing all the bones.
3 Mash the potatoes with the butter, milk, parsley, lemon zest and salt and pepper. Mix in the flaked fish. With floured hands, shape into 8 round cakes. Beat the egg in a shallow bowl. Coat each cake with the egg, then the dried breadcrumbs and leave in the fridge for about 30 minutes.
4 Heat the oil in a large frying pan over medium heat and fry the fishcakes for 6–8 minutes, turning halfway through cooking. Drain on kitchen paper. Alternatively, grill them under a preheated grill for approximately 8 minutes, turning halfway through.

Sea breeze

Grapefruit juice gives you a vitamin C boost and cranberry juice contains powerful antioxidants to protect you against heart disease. It also has a beneficial effect on bladder and urinary tract infections.

MAKES 2 DRINKS
50ml (2fl oz) vodka
75ml (3fl oz) cranberry juice
75ml (3fl oz) grapefruit juice
10 cracked ice cubes
2 lime slices to decorate

1 Put the vodka, cranberry and grapefruit juices into a cocktail shaker with the ice cubes. Shake briefly and pour into two tall glasses.
2 Decorate each with a lime slice and serve with a straw.

Lovers' dream

Blackberries and raspberries are two of the richest sources of vitamin C and folate (both of which help protect you against heart disease) of all fruit. They're also packed with anthocyanins, which help combat free radicals, strengthen collagen in the skin and reduce wrinkles.

MAKES 2 DRINKS
4 large raspberries
2 large blackberries
1/2 bottle of champagne

1 Take two champagne glasses and place two raspberries and a blackberry in each glass. Crush them with the flat end of a teaspoon.
2 Slowly top up with champagne.

New year, new you

Christmas is a time of giving and receiving. Giving presents and receiving extra calories thanks to the rich foods, fine wines and lack of exercise that seem to go hand-in-hand with the festive season. That's why a whole different approach to food and drink in January can get your body *and* your mind back into shape, ready for the new year and the new you.

Let me stress ... this is *not* a detox diet. Personally, I hate the concept of detoxing. The aim of the 'New Year, New You' plan is to get you back on track after the Christmas season of over-eating and drinking. It will help improve your skin tone and digestion which took a battering through December. So you'll regain your energy and enjoy clearer, more youthful skin, improved sleep, greater mental clarity and a more efficient immune system. And you might even lose some weight too. Mentally, it is a great way of getting you into thinking about healthy eating habits which can last all year round.

⟶ You should still be drinking at least 2 litres (4½ pints) of filtered or mineral water a day. If that fell by the wayside over Christmas, make sure you get back into the habit as soon as you can.

⟶ The party season's over so it's back to regular meals and healthy food. Eat sensibly and regularly.

⟶ Don't avoid fats; you may be carrying a few extra pounds thanks to all the mince pies but fat-free diets aren't the way to lose them. Use sparingly but include extra-virgin olive oil or flaxseed oil as a dressing or to cook with. 'Good' fat carries important vitamins round the body.

Restore, renourish, replenish

Breakfast

···> Start the day with warm water and freshly squeezed lemon juice to wake up your digestive system and to get your metabolism going.

···> Follow that with some juice. Juicing is a great way to get your daily intake of fruit and veg and it can help the detox process too. Fresh apple juice (cleansing tonic) or spinach juice (which acts as an eliminator) are ideal.

···> Don't skip breakfast – have a bowl of porridge. Oats help flush away toxins, release energy slowly to prevent cravings and lower cholesterol in blood.

···> Alternatively, only eat raw fruit and veg in the morning. This helps the liver's natural detoxification process which is at its most active between midnight and midday.

···> The riper the fruit, the more antioxidant vitamins and minerals it contains.

···> If you prefer a smoothie to start the day, whiz up a couple of bananas, a tablespoon of peanut butter, a small pot of plain live yogurt and half a teaspoon of cinnamon.

···> Make sure your diet is rich in vitamin C which supports the liver detox process.

Lunch

···> Vegetable soup is an efficient way to absorb essential nutrients. You can add your favourite veggies to a home-made stock. A mixture of green beans, courgettes, celery, garlic, parsley, ginger, cayenne pepper, thyme and rosemary boosts the immune system and cleanses the liver at the same time. The herbs are a wonderful pick-me-up too.

···> Ensure you are eating vegetables like broccoli, red cabbage, carrots, cauliflower, kale, pumpkin, spinach and sweet potato; they're full of beta carotenes. They're also packed with antioxidants and are extremely effective at helping the liver detox the body.

···> Include leeks in your meals. Eating a leek is a bit like eating a gentle brush. The long fibres pick up impurities as they pass through the digestive system, taking all the bad stuff with them. Rich in potassium, leeks are an effective diuretic and have similar health-giving properties to garlic and onions.

···> Sardines or baked beans on wholemeal toast: easy and quick to prepare.

···> Whip up some guacamole. The avocados are full of vitamin E and antioxidants, the chillies give the circulation a boost and the red peppers are full of antioxidants.

⋯⋗ Chop up some red and yellow peppers, carrots, cauliflower and celery to dip in the guacamole and to nibble throughout the day.

⋯⋗ Have a drink of ginger tea. It is a great stimulant, speeds up the circulation and helps eliminate toxins. It's a tasty and warming drink to enjoy in the depths of winter.

Dinner

⋯⋗ Plan ahead. Work out a week's evening meals and make sure you add variety. Choose a different lean protein for each night: skinless chicken or turkey breast; salmon, mackerel or tuna; and eat with slow-release carbohydrates such as brown rice or a baked potato.

⋯⋗ For a change, end your day on an egg. Whip up a tasty frittata.

⋯⋗ Make sure you add at least one vegetable to your evening meal. Again, don't stick to one or two all the time. Mix them up and have different ones with each meal.

⋯⋗ Alternatively, make a tasty ratatouille. With courgettes, aubergines, peppers, garlic, tomatoes, olive oil and herbs, this can be a great accompaniment to a main meal or a dish on its own.

⋯⋗ A little garlic will go a long way. Thanks to the sulphur compounds found in allicin (the antioxidant that is released when you crush a fresh clove), garlic is great at replenishing our immune systems. Cooking the garlic doesn't lessen the benefits; just let the bulbs sit for a few minutes after you've peeled them before using them.

⋯⋗ Really cut down on the booze. Yes, there are advantages to the odd glass of red wine but your liver's probably taken a battering over Christmas. Give it a rest and let it get on with what it's designed to do: eliminating harmful substances like toxins from your body to maintain optimum health. And as an added bonus, if you give up drinking in the evening, you could lose 4.5kg (9½ lb) a year.

SALT IS GOOD . . .
. . . if you add a cup of sea salt to your bath to stimulate your skin, give it a healthy glow and help rid it of toxins. You can also mix some salt with almond oil and massage it into damp skin to act as a natural exfoliator.

Restorative recipes

As well as the recipes that follow, try these suggestions:

⋯⇢ Pumpkin/sweet potato soup

⋯⇢ Garlic soup

⋯⇢ Chickpea casserole – full of fibre, B vitamins and minerals which is great for the skin at this – or any – time of the year.

⋯⇢ Chicken casserole with garlic, onions, celery, mushrooms, thyme. Chicken contains low-fat protein, iron, zinc, vitamin B6; onions, garlic and mushrooms are immune-boosters. Herbs add flavour without having to resort to too much salt.

⋯⇢ Guacamole

⋯⇢ Ratatouille

Chicken casserole with lentils and leeks

Chicken is a low-fat source of protein as well as B vitamins, iron and zinc. In this healthy casserole, it is slow-cooked with Puy lentils (which provide a good balance of protein and complex carbohydrates as well as soluble fibre, iron, B vitamins, zinc and magnesium) and leeks, which are great natural diuretic foods.

SERVES 2
15ml (1 tbsp) extra-virgin olive oil
2 chicken breasts
125g (4oz) leeks, trimmed and thickly sliced
1 small onion, peeled and sliced
125g (4oz) carrots, peeled and sliced
2 sage leaves, roughly chopped
60g (2oz) Puy lentils
250ml (9fl oz) chicken stock
A little low-sodium salt and freshly ground black pepper
2 tbsp chopped fresh parsley

1 Pre-heat the oven to 190°C/375°F/Gas mark 5.
2 Heat the oil in a flameproof casserole dish on the hob and brown the chicken. Add the leeks, onion and carrots and continue cooking for a few minutes. Add the sage, lentils and stock and bring to the boil. Season with the low-sodium salt and black pepper.
3 Cover and simmer in the oven for 1 hour or until the chicken is very tender, stirring halfway through cooking. Stir in the chopped parsley just before serving.

Caldo verde

This healthy version of the classic Portuguese dish is made with curly kale and Savoy cabbage, both of which are packed with immunity-enhancing vitamin C, beta carotene, folate and iron. Don't discard the outer green leaves – they contain up to 50 times the vitamins as the inner pale ones.

SERVES 2
15ml (1 tbsp) extra-virgin olive oil
1/2 onion, peeled and chopped
1 garlic clove, peeled and crushed
225g (8oz) potatoes, peeled and diced
500 ml (17fl oz) vegetable stock
225g (8oz) mixture of curly kale and Savoy cabbage, finely shredded
A little low-sodium salt and freshly ground black pepper, to taste

1 Heat the olive oil in a large heavy-based pan and cook the onion, garlic and potatoes over a moderate heat for about 5 minutes. Add the stock and shredded greens, bring to the boil, and then simmer for 20 minutes until the vegetables are tender.
2 Remove half of the soup and liquidize using a hand blender or conventional blender. Return to the pan and stir well. Add a little more water if necessary to thin to a soupy consistency and reheat for a minute or two until piping hot.
3 Season with low-sodium salt and plenty of black pepper. Ladle into soup bowls, pour a drizzle of olive oil over each one and serve.

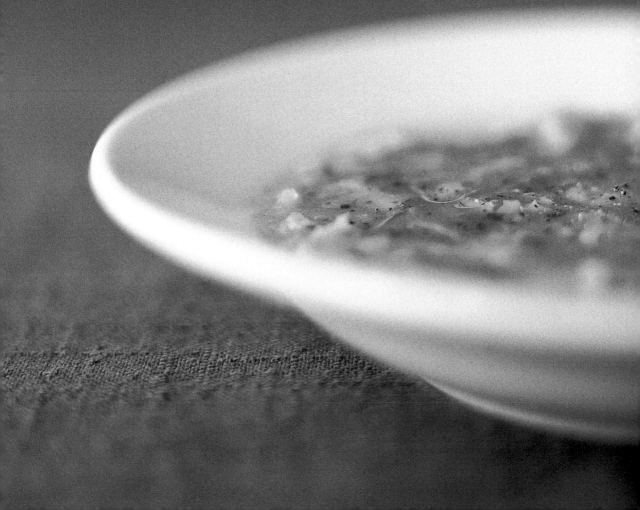

'Soup puts the heart at ease, calms down the violence of hunger, eliminates the tension of the day, and awakens and refines the appetite.' AUGUST ESCOFFIER

Holiday countdown

You want to go away on your well-deserved holiday feeling firm, toned, glowing with energy and looking fantastic. So, naturally, you want to get in shape before you go.

I believe that following a healthy eating plan regularly can keep you looking youthful, sleek and feeling great, so I don't generally advocate going on a diet as a long-term solution. However, I do appreciate that now and again it doesn't hurt to concentrate on shedding a few pounds before a big event. A youthful look is *not* about not being underweight – it's exactly the opposite and in fact being too thin can add years to a person. If you are a size and weight that you feel happy with, your self-esteem and energy levels are high and that's the kind of state of mind that can make you look and feel ten years younger.

First of all, be realistic with yourself and *don't* crash diet. That will make you feel lousy, is really bad for your skin and you probably won't achieve the desired effect in the end anyway. If you lose too much weight too quickly, the layer of fat that sits just below the surface of your skin will disappear as well; it's that fat that plumps out your wrinkles and gives the skin its youthful appearance.

Losing weight is quite simple really. You need to eat fewer calories than you are using. If you do little or no exercise, think about doing three 20–30 minute sessions a week to help you shed those pounds. If you already work out, either increase it to four or five times a week or reduce your calorie intake – but be sensible about it.

'Sometimes I get to a point when I think I should lose a bit of tummy for the beach. Then I'll be careful and I won't have pudding for a few weeks or I'll do more riding.' **JODIE KIDD, MODEL**

Eating for a holiday body

→ Put smaller portions on smaller plates. You're eating less but your plate still looks full! For example, reducing the amount of chicken from 150g (5oz) to 75g (3oz) can shave off around 200 calories.

→ Avoid too many starchy carbohydrates and stock up on fruit, veg and fluids. You want to get rid of excess fluids that can bloat your tummy, thighs and bottom. Fruit and veg are also full of healthy antioxidants which will have a positive anti-ageing effect on skin.

→ Forget worrying about food combining and whether you can mix proteins with starch. I disagree with the whole concept. Our bodies are highly sophisticated machines that digest and absorb nutrients at different points along our digestive tract. You're aiming for a healthy balance of great anti-ageing foods. Look at chapter three for a list of fab foods.

→ Say goodbye to coffee and tea with milk and hello to green and white tea. Research from Nottingham University has shown that adding milk to tea reduces the amount of anti-ageing antioxidants you absorb from it. Ordinary tea and coffee are diuretics so encourage our bodies to eliminate water. This builds up the toxic overload in our bodies, making our skin dull and puffy which is very ageing. Green and white tea, as well as being packed full of antioxidants and flavonoids which preserve the structure of the skin, boost your metabolism and help to burn up extra calories. Drinking five cups a day burns 4 per cent more calories and lowers the body's absorption of non-essential fats by as much as 30 per cent.

→ Dandelion tea is great at flushing out toxins by stimulating the liver and breaking down fat. Dandelion is full of vitamins A and C which are wonderful for skin. The French love dandelion salad. If you can't get the leaves, try the tea which is ideal for reducing puffiness and cellulite – just think of how good you're going to look in that bikini!

→ Keep drinking water. You need to keep your water levels topped up to ensure your metabolism is working effectively. Water hydrates skin, acting like a moisturizer to plump it up and keep it looking fresh.

→ Eat foods that are rich in serotonin (such as milk or bananas). Serotonin controls our appetite so the more you have in your diet, the less likely you are to overeat. If you can control your appetite, you also balance your blood sugar levels and insulin production. High blood sugar and insulin ultimately destroy collagen which means wrinkly, tough skin; while the excess sugar is stored as fat.

Breakfast

···❭ Kick-start your day and your metabolism with a mug of warm water with a squeeze of lemon juice. You'll flush out toxins and lose weight (you burn up 12 calories for every glass of water you drink).

···❭ Then, breakfast – *the* most important meal of the day and a great way to wake up your metabolism so don't skip it. Why not go to work on an egg? Protein and fat in eggs help stop mid-morning snacking. So you eat less for lunch. Research has shown that if you start the day with scrambled eggs you can end up eating 430 fewer calories over the day. Eggs have all the essential amino acids in the right proportions and are full of Omega-3 fatty acids and vitamin A.

···❭ Or choose a pot of low-fat yogurt with a handful of berries sprinkled over the top. Finish off with an apple. The berries and apples provide antioxidants, flavonoids and polyphenols which combat the ageing free radicals; while the yogurt ensures that your digestion is working efficiently, processing all the vitamins and minerals so they continue to replenish and maintain your body, keeping it looking young and healthy.

Firming fruit

···❭ Fruit contains fibre which will help fill you up and contains vitamin C which is great for your skin.

···❭ Apples and celery have high levels of leptin which help the body metabolize fat cells and reduce fat storage in subcutaneous layers.

···❭ Add a grapefruit to your daily diet to help you lose weight. Studies have found that people who eat grapefruit lose weight faster (NB grapefruit juice can react with some medication so check with your GP). It contains pectin which helps your digestion and your circulation. Pink grapefruit can give you a youthful pink glow too; they contain more beta carotenes than any other kind so they're great for your complexion.

Lunch

···❭ Try a bowl of healthy vegetable soup. Research shows that eating soup before your meal will help you to lose weight. Sprinkle some flax seeds over the soup; they're full of Omega-3 and -6 fatty acids which are vital for healthy skin, nails and hair.

- Alternatively, fill a wholemeal pitta bread with 2 tbsp of low-fat hummus and eat with loads of crunchy bright crudités (red and orange peppers, sticks of celery, cucumber, carrots – full of antioxidants to fight those damaging free radicals).

- Or try a salad of chickpeas and tomatoes (see page 280). Chickpeas are full of soluble fibre which gives a steady flow of energy and keeps your blood sugar levels stable, so they're great for maintaining healthy skin because there's no extra sugar to damage the collagen levels or end up as extra fat where you don't want it.

- Eat brown – consuming brown, complex carbohydrates cuts down our desire to eat sugary, fattening foods. Brown foods are full of healthy fibre which keeps you regular and stops your entire system from becoming sluggish and slow; this in turn means no added cellulite, healthy-looking skin and bags of energy – great for looking and feeling young.

DID YOU KNOW?
450g (1lb) of weight is equal to 3,500 calories so you need to cut back by about 500 calories a day to lose 450g (1lb) a week. » Overeating fatty food, especially saturated fat, prompts the production of galanin which increases our desire for more food.

Evening meal

- Have a light evening meal, such as grilled chicken or fish with some steamed vegetables. It's not too fattening, you'll digest it easily and you'll sleep better. The protein in the meat is wonderful for maintaining smooth skin and great muscle tone; the vegetables are full of anti-ageing antioxidants.

- Have a cut-off point in the evening when you stop eating. Night-time nibbles can add on an amazing number of calories if you're not careful.

- Before going to bed, drink 500ml (17fl oz) of cold water; it increases your metabolic rate by about 30 per cent and plumps up your skin.

- You need to get a good night's sleep. If you're getting less than six hours, your body won't be burning off sugar as efficiently as it should and that means it will be stored as fat. It also leaves you looking run down and tired which can add years to your looks.

- Try not to eat carbs after 5pm; this will help you enjoy some quality sleep.

Holiday countdown recipes

Chickpea and cherry tomato salad

This protein-rich salad can be varied by using ready-bought marinated artichoke hearts or aubergines instead of the peppers, and substituting other fresh herbs for the basil and parsley. Chickpeas are an excellent source of fibre, protein and iron. They contain fructo-oligosaccharides, a type of fibre that maintains healthy gut flora.

SERVES 2
225g (8oz) cooked or canned chickpeas, rinsed and drained
125g (4oz) ready-bought marinated peppers
125g (4oz) cherry tomatoes, halved
3 or 4 spring onions, sliced
Small handful of fresh basil leaves
Small handful of fresh parsley, chopped
Freshly ground black pepper

FOR THE DRESSING:
30ml (2 tbsp) extra-virgin olive oil
10ml (2 tsp) lemon juice
1.25ml ($^1/_2$ tsp) Dijon mustard
1 small garlic clove, peeled and crushed

1 Put the chickpeas, peppers, cherry tomatoes and spring onions in a bowl and combine well.
2 Make the dressing by placing the ingredients into a screw-top glass jar and shaking well.
3 Pour the dressing over the salad. Add the herbs and black pepper and mix together well. Chill and serve.

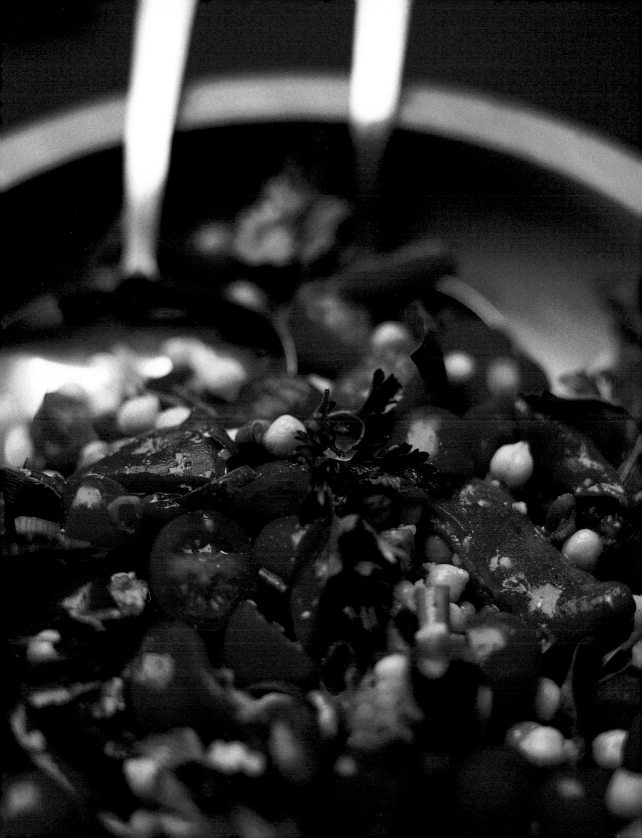

Mango and strawberry fruit salad with lime

This simple, aromatic combination of fresh fruits looks stunning. Mangoes are the best fruit source of the antioxidant beta carotene, which helps promote healthy skin and improve its elasticity. It also provides vitamin C, vitamin E and potassium. Strawberries are super-rich in vitamin C, which is good for strengthening blood vessels and protecting the skin against free-radical damage.

SERVES 2
1 small ripe mango
225g (8oz) strawberries
Grated zest and juice of 1 lime
10ml (2 tsp) acacia honey

1 Slice through the mango either side of the stone, then cut the flesh into cubes. Wash, hull and halve the strawberries. Place all the fruit in a serving bowl.
2 Grate the zest from the lime and add to the fruit. Squeeze the juice, then put in a small saucepan with the honey. Heat gently, stirring, just until the honey has dissolved. Allow to cool.
3 Pour the cooled lime juice mixture over the fruit and toss gently.

Youthful snacks

I don't snack between meals. I believe that three good meals a day is enough to keep you satisfied. However, I appreciate that not everyone can go without between meals.

If that's the case, then I think it's better to eat six smaller meals a day rather than try and go cold turkey, failing and ending up eating rubbish. If you eat consistently, your metabolism will get into a routine and the sudden wild appetite swings will disappear.

Snack attack

Next time you find yourself wanting to eat between meals, ask yourself if you are actually hungry or are you just thirsty, bored, tired or fed up? Snacks are often nothing to do with being genuinely hungry and everything to do with our state of mind. Be honest. Have you ever snacked at work just to have a break from your job? Has it become a habit to buy the evening paper and a bar of chocolate on the way home? Have you grazed on sweets in the car on long journeys? If you answer yes to any (or all!), then you're not alone. The trick is to re-educate your mind *and* your stomach. Next time the mid-morning munchies bite, have a glass of water before you do anything else. Then see how hungry you really are. You may find you actually lose the urge to snack.

In the meantime, if you really do need to graze on something, make sure that it's healthy and, more importantly, youthful. Keep the snacks handy in case you do get the urge to eat. On the next page you'll find a few suggestions.

Vegetables

⇢ Chop up carrots, red peppers, cherry tomatoes – a great source of antioxidants. Carrots contain carotenoids which protect against the damaging effect of sunlight on skin; red peppers and tomatoes contain lycopene which slows down skin degeneration. Eat them on their own or dip them in hummus. The chickpeas and tahini in hummus are full of vitamin E which is great for your skin and they provide protein, iron and folic acid. Or take a pot of plain natural yogurt and add a spoonful of Manuka honey and have that as a dip. Yogurt is good for your digestion and honey adds a sweetness without the calories and ageing effects of refined sugar.

⇢ Take a flask of vegetable soup to work. A good home-made stock with chopped-up vegetables will fill you with vitamins and minerals. For something more substantial, add protein in the form of cooked diced chicken or canned beans (protein is essential for the production of collagen, enzymes, muscles, hormones and nerves). Make up a large quantity and freeze the excess in individual portions.

⇢ Roasted vegetables with a drizzle of olive oil and balsamic vinegar taste just as good cold as they do hot. Cook up a large batch and keep some for the next day. Olive oil is a good source of Omega-9 fatty acids which keep cell membranes moisturized, helping to reduce wrinkles and maintain a youthful complexion.

Fruit

⇢ Dried apricots, figs, prunes and raisins make handy snacks, but they can be high in sugar so only nibble on two or three. Drink a glass of water while nibbling them to help the fibre swell and make you feel full.

⇢ A banana and a low-fat natural yogurt are an ideal mid-morning or afternoon snack. Bananas have been called the original fast food and, unlike most of today's 'fast foods', they're actually good for you.

⇢ Make a fruit shake (mix fresh fruit with low-fat yogurt or skimmed milk).

⇢ Wholewheat blueberry and walnut muffins for a healthy treat now and again (see the recipe on page 286). Blueberries contain resveratrol, a flavonoid which seems to decrease the ageing of DNA in the mito-chondria, the energy plant of the cell which is so good for keeping skin looking young. Walnuts contain protein, iron and calcium.

Nuts and seeds

⋯▹ Brazil nuts or almonds make great power snacks. They're high in protein so are good for giving you an energy boost if you're beginning to flag and the essential fatty acids are great for your skin.

⋯▹ Peanuts – not the salty, oily kind... just the nuts. A Harvard University study of 83,000 women found that those who ate 150g (5oz) of peanuts a week had healthier hearts and were thinner than those who didn't.

⋯▹ Pumpkin seeds – lots of zinc and vitamin E which are vital for healthy, moisturized skin.

Sandwiches

⋯▹ Go for the wholemeal option. Wholemeal contains the essential amino acids, vitamin E, B vitamins, zinc, iron, copper and fibre. Silica is found in whole grains; it helps the skin store moisture and so reduces wrinkles and skin problems.

⋯▹ When buying sandwiches, look at the label to help pick the healthiest option. Choose a sandwich that is less than 20g fat, less than 2g salt, less than 5g saturated fat.

Biscuits

⋯▹ Don't get excited, I'm not talking custard creams here. Try a couple of oatcakes, topped with a teaspoon of peanut butter or hummus. Oats contain a type of fibre called beta-glucans which will slow down sugar absorption so you don't get sudden highs and lows; good for appetite control and keeping your blood sugar levels balanced. Peanut butter is full of iron (which transports oxygen to every cell), magnesium (for strong bones and teeth) and zinc (essential for the production of collagen).

⋯▹ If you're not keen on peanut butter, spread your oatcakes with some reduced-fat soft cheese – a good source of calcium which is vital for the skin, bones and teeth.

⋯▹ Try rice cakes with low-fat cottage cheese and a drizzle of Manuka honey.

SNACKS TO AVOID
The bad kinds are full of salt, sugar and fat which have no nutritional value, do absolutely nothing for your health or your skin and can cause you to lurch from sugar-low to high and back again in a very short time. Steer clear of crisps, sweets and sweet biscuits.

Snacktime recipes

Salmon and spinach wrap

This wrap is a great way of adding two anti-ageing foods to your diet. Salmon is rich in Omega-3s, which help strengthen skin from within, improving its elasticity and reducing the formation of wrinkles. Spinach is full of iron, vitamin C, folate and beta carotene, all of which give skin a nutritional boost.

SERVES 1
50g (2oz) salmon (poached or tinned)
15ml (1 tbsp) lemon juice
Freshly ground black pepper
15ml (1 tbsp) reduced calorie mayonnaise
40g (1¹/₂ oz) baby spinach leaves
40g (1¹/₂ oz) cucumber, sliced
1 large or 2 small tortilla wraps

1 Flake the salmon and mix with the lemon juice, black pepper and mayonnaise. Place the salmon mixture, baby spinach and cucumber along the centre of the wrap. Fold and roll the wrap to secure the filling.
2 Cut into two or four pieces, depending on the size of the wrap.

Blueberry and walnut muffins

This recipe is a delicious way of adding antioxidant-rich blueberries to your diet. These muffins are lower in fat than ordinary muffins, providing mostly healthy monounsaturated fats, higher in fibre and rich in vitamins.

MAKES 12 MUFFINS
125g (4oz) self-raising white flour
125g (4oz) self-raising wholemeal flour
60g (2oz) sugar
45ml (3 tbsp) rapeseed or sunflower oil
1 egg
250ml (8fl oz) apple purée
5ml (1 tsp) vanilla extract
200ml (7fl oz) skimmed milk
125g (4 oz) fresh blueberries (or 85g/3oz dried blueberries)
60g (2oz) walnut pieces

1 Pre-heat the oven to 200°C/400°F/Gas mark 6. Line a 12-hole muffin tin with paper cases.
2 In a bowl, mix together the flours and sugar. In a separate bowl, mix together the oil, egg, apple purée, vanilla extract and milk, then pour into the flour mixture. Stir until just combined. Gently fold in the blueberries and walnuts.
3 Spoon the mixture into the paper cases (about two-thirds full) and bake for about 20 minutes until the muffins are risen and golden.

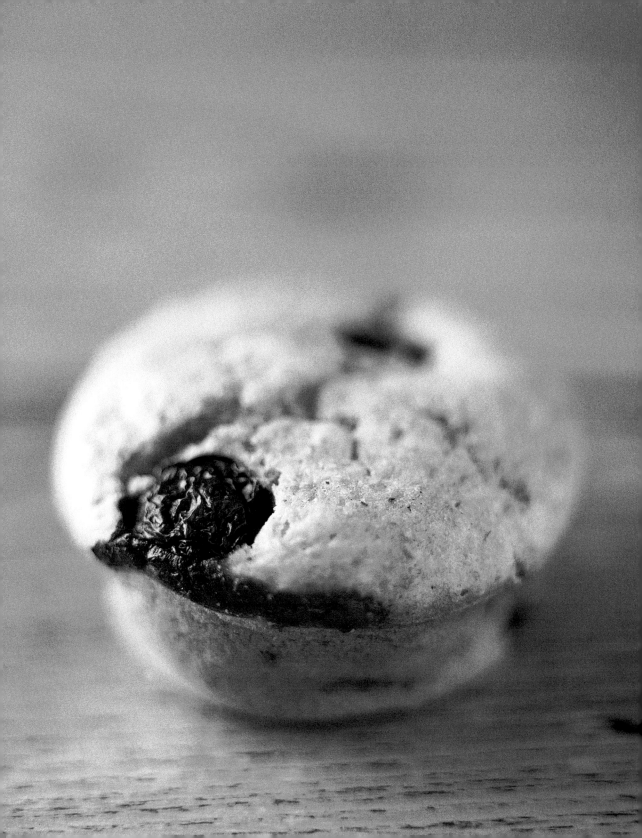

The wrinkle-zapping dinner party

We all like to push the boat out for a special occasion but that doesn't mean you have to eat food that isn't going to do you any good or gorge yourself stupid. Hopefully, you will have realized from reading this book that there are fantastic foods that look and taste great *and* will make you look younger too.

As you will know by now, 'healthy' food doesn't have to be boring, dull, colourless and tasteless. And a wrinkle-zapping dinner party, using the suggestions that follow, is a great opportunity to show off your culinary skills and enjoy some great anti-ageing foods at the same time.

Drinks

You don't have to restrict your guests to two small glasses of wine during the evening. But you don't want to encourage over-indulgence either. Wine is a perfect accompaniment to a meal.

⇢ Tall thin glasses give the impression that they hold more than short ones. Studies have shown that people drink 20 per cent more from stubbier glasses. If you use tall narrow glasses people think they're drinking more than they actually are and won't feel deprived.

⇢ Make sure you have bottles of water and glasses for your guests throughout the meal; they'll be encouraged to drink less alcohol.

⇢ Water also suppresses the appetite so people won't overeat.

⇢ Red wine is the best kind of wine to drink. It contains the powerful protective antioxidant resveratrol which slows down the ageing of the DNA in the mitochondria, the energy plant of the cell. The best grapes for maximum benefit are Cabernet Sauvignon, Merlot and Pinot Noir.

Nibbles and starters

---> Offer bowls of olives and nuts because they're rich in Omega-3, -6 and -9s which keep our skin cells supple and flexible, reduce wrinkles and have powerful anti-inflammatory properties.

---> Fresh crudités are a tasty start to a meal. They're not too filling and they have amazing anti-ageing properties. Beta carotene is found in bright yellow and deep green vegetables such as carrots and peppers. In the body, beta carotene is converted to retinol (vitamin A) which neutralizes free radicals and protects our skin's cell structure, slowing down the effect of ageing. Lycopene is a naturally occurring red pigment in food (tomatoes, red peppers) which helps to slow down and prevent cells from ageing.

---> Serve the crudités with salsa, hummus, tapenade and/or guacamole. The dips contain either tomatoes, garlic and onions (full of vitamin C to fight damaging free radicals and to boost the intake of oxygen to cells to keep the skin looking healthy), protein, essential for healthy cells and collagen production, from chickpeas and tahini, Omega-9 (essential fatty acids) from the olive oil and olives; herbs, such as basil (which helps break down food to allow absorption of nutrients) and parsley (full of vitamin C and great for ridding impurities and toxins).

---> Soup is a great starter for a meal. It won't fill your guests up too much, it's easy to prepare and get ready (so ideal from the hostess' point of view) and, depending on what sort you serve, can be extremely healthy. Avoid creamy soups. Go for soups that have super foods as their main ingredient. For example, asparagus accelerates the production of new cells and helps eliminate waste from the body. Borsch has beetroot as its main ingredient, a great source of beta carotene (an antioxidant) and potassium (which helps remove toxins by stimulating the kidneys and prevents skin from looking dull and sluggish). If making chicken soup, the breast meat is low in saturated fat, it's a good source of protein and also contains B vitamins, iron and zinc: all of which help replenish and repair the skin cells.

---> To finish off the presentation, use a little yogurt, rather than cream. Yogurt is a good source of protein, vitamins A, B, D and E, calcium, potassium (which helps eliminate waste) and phosphorus (which helps the body repair itself and maintain good bones and teeth).

---> Alternatively, sprinkle the soup with some flaxseeds which are a powerful source of Omega-3 and -6 essential fatty acids (absolutely brilliant for great looking skin).

Main course

Something fishy

Fish is top of the class when it comes to anti-ageing properties. Of all the main course foods you could choose from, fish should be first choice.

···◊ Wild salmon has three times the amount of Omega-3 oils as farmed varieties, higher antioxidant levels and less fat.

···◊ Salmon also contains copper (which helps produce melanin that protects our skin against the sun) and zinc which helps keep our collagen supply at maximum, reducing the effect of wrinkles and sun damage on our skin.

···◊ Salmon, and fish like it, is a great source of protein which the body breaks down into essential amino acids. These amino acids are vital in the manufacture of collagen.

···◊ DMAE is brain food as well and helps to improve memory and clarify thoughts – which should make the conversation around the dinner table sparkle.

···◊ Seafood contains selenium which slows down the ageing process and zinc which is essential for collagen production.

···◊ Choose from: salmon, mackerel, trout, sardines, tuna, anchovies which all contain high levels of essential fatty acids. See pages 225–229 for more info.

'The flesh of fish – especially salmon – contains DMAE, a powerful antioxidant. DMAE is your magic bullet for great skin tone, keeping your face firm and contoured. It prevents and reverses what is clinically known as "anatomical loss of position", commonly known as sagging.' DR NICHOLAS PERRICONE

Game for a meal

Wild game is full of flavour but low in fat compared with farmed meat. It comes with the benefit of no added hormones, steroids or antibiotics and has a great flavour.

⋯⋗ Game is a rich source of selenium (an antioxidant which helps remove free radicals from the body to protect against premature ageing), zinc (which protects and repairs DNA) and iron (used to make haemoglobin which carries oxygen to every cell in the body; healthy cells maintain skin texture and suppleness).

Vital vegetables

Just look through the super foods (see page 102) to see how many vegetables make the list. They are full of powerful antioxidants, great at protecting our skins against damaging free radicals and helping to preserve our youthful looks. My top three are:

⋯⋗ Carrots – we can absorb 13 times more of the antioxidant beta carotene from carrots if they are simply served with a knob of butter or stir-fried in a little olive oil (great source of Omega-9 fatty acids).

⋯⋗ Broccoli – just a single serving contains 200 per cent of the recommended daily amount of vitamin C and calcium. It's also a wonderful source of beta carotene which is essential for the reproduction and maintenance of epithelial tissue which keeps skin smooth and supple. As a veg, it's very low in fat and calories.

⋯⋗ Sweet potatoes are also full of beta carotene which is stored in the fat layer of our skin and protects against the damage from the sun's ultraviolet rays.

Puddings and cheese

⇢ A big bowl of fruit salad or seasonal berries can look great and taste amazing. A fruit compote (the fruits will depend on the season) is also a healthy way to finish the meal. In the winter, choose from prunes, pears, plums, apples, figs, dried apricots; in the summer, the world's your oyster – go for strawberries, raspberries, blueberries, mango, guava, pineapple. Skip the cream; offer guests a dollop of Greek yogurt instead.

⇢ Soak some prunes (extremely high levels of antioxidants) in Armagnac. Serve with thick live natural yogurt (good for the digestion and an excellent source of calcium).

⇢ If you would prefer a slightly more sinful pudding, go for one that contains dark chocolate. Dark chocolate (with at least 70 per cent cocoa solids) has a protective effect on the brain and contains anti-ageing antioxidants called phenols.

⇢ And finally, the cheese board. Cheese is full of calcium for strong bones and teeth which helps to preserve that youthful look; there's nothing more ageing than frail bones and bad teeth. Be careful which cheese you choose because some have a higher fat content than others. Edam and feta are low in fat and any cheese made from goat's or sheep's milk is going to be lower in fat and lactose than one made from cow's milk. Serve with oatcakes (which help preserve the quality of your skin by keeping blood sugar levels balanced) and a bunch of red grapes (which contain anthocyanins, important antioxidant flavonoids).

'A dinner which ends without cheese is like a beautiful woman with only one eye.'

JEAN-ANTHELME BRILLAT-SAVARIN

Dinner party menus

As well as the two three-course menus that follow, try these suggestions for a dinner party to hold back the years:

Starters
···⟩ Soups
···⟩ Prawn cocktail: rather than cover prawns with sauce, chop a handful of cherry tomatoes. Add chopped cucumber and spring onions, 1 tbsp chopped dill, 2 tsp each of lime juice and olive oil.
···⟩ Roasted red pepper tarts – rich in vitamins A and C, folic acid and potassium.

Main course
···⟩ Venison casserole/steaks
···⟩ Salmon

Puddings
···⟩ Figs with goat's cheese, drizzled with honey and toasted pine nuts – lots of iron, potassium, beta carotene, fibre and energy.
···⟩ Green tea and apple granita
···⟩ Fruit compote
···⟩ Poached pears

Menu One

Asparagus and avocado salad with walnuts

Asparagus is rich in folate and vitamin E and contains a special type of fibre – fructo-oligosaccharides – that benefits your digestive system. Avocados are excellent sources of monounsaturated oils that help to keep your heart healthy and also do wonders for your skin.

SERVES 4
225g (8oz) asparagus spears
2 avocados
30ml (2 tbsp) lemon juice
2–3 handfuls salad leaves, eg rocket, watercress, lettuce
85g (3oz) walnuts, lightly toasted

FOR THE DRESSING:
15ml (1 tbsp) walnut oil
15ml (1 tbsp) olive oil
10ml (2 tsp) cider vinegar
5ml (1 tsp) lemon juice

1 Trim the asparagus spears. Steam for 3 minutes until they are still quite crunchy. Drain and allow them to cool.
2 Cut the avocados in half, remove the stone and peel. Dice the flesh and toss immediately in the lemon juice to prevent it from going brown.
3 Remove the avocado from the lemon juice and mix with the asparagus spears. Divide the salad leaves onto 4 small plates and arrange the asparagus and avocado over. Place the dressing ingredients in a screw-top jar and shake well to combine. Drizzle over the salad and scatter over the walnuts.

Chicken breasts filled with prunes, almonds and wild rice

This impressive chicken dish is filled with prunes, one of the richest fruit sources of antioxidant nutrients and fibre, as well as almonds (excellent for calcium and zinc) and wild rice (contains B vitamins). Prunes also contain hydroxycinnamic acid, a powerful antioxidant that helps combat free radical damage associated with premature ageing.

SERVES 4
150g (5oz) wild rice
4 chicken breasts, skinless
8 soft ready-to-eat prunes, chopped
25g (1oz) almonds, lightly toasted and chopped
25g (1oz) raisins
30ml (2 tbsp) parsley, finely chopped
2 garlic cloves, peeled and crushed
A little low-sodium salt and freshly ground black pepper

1 Pre-heat the oven to 200°C/400°F/Gas mark 6. Cook the wild rice according to the packet instructions.
2 Meanwhile, place the chicken breasts on a chopping board and, using a sharp knife, cut a pocket into them along the length of the sides. Mix together the cooked rice, prunes, almonds, raisins, parsley, garlic, salt and pepper. Fill each chicken pocket with the rice and prune mixture. Close the pocket and secure with two cocktail sticks.
3 Heat the oil in a non-stick pan and cook the chicken breasts for 2 minutes over a moderate heat, turning to seal all over. Transfer to an ovenproof dish; pour over 100ml (3^1/$_2$ fl oz) water and cook in the oven for 10–12 minutes until the chicken is cooked and tender. Remove from the oven. Serve with a leafy salad, ideally watercress and rocket.

Vanilla pears with cherry compote

The delicate flavours of the poached pears complement perfectly the sharpness of the cherry compote. Conference pears work particularly well in this recipe. Pears are also a good source of hydroxycinnamic acid, as well as potassium, fibre and reasonable quantities of vitamin C.

SERVES 4
4 ripe pears
60ml (4 tbsp) clear honey
1 strip lemon peel
1 strip orange peel
Juice of $1/2$ lemon
1 vanilla pod, split lengthways

FOR THE CHERRY COMPOTE:
60ml (2fl oz) water
60g (2oz) caster sugar
200g (7oz) canned black cherries, drained
OR 60ml (4 tbsp) ready-made cherry compote

1 Peel the whole pears carefully with a vegetable peeler, making them look as smooth as possible. You can leave the stalks on. Put them in a small saucepan so they fit snugly together.
2 Cover with water. Add the honey, the lemon and orange peel and the lemon juice. Scrape the seeds from the vanilla pod into the pan and add the pod itself. Bring the pan to the boil, reduce the heat, cover and simmer for about 15 minutes (depending on the size of the pears) until just cooked. Allow to cool in the cooking liquor. Remove the pears. Heat the remaining liquor to a rapid boil and reduce until the syrup has thickened.
3 Meanwhile, make the cherry compote. Place the water and caster sugar in a saucepan. Place over a moderate heat and gently warm until the sugar dissolves into the water. Add the cherries and gently cook for 2–3 minutes.
4 Place the pears on individual serving plates. Spoon a little syrup over each pear and serve with a spoonful of cherry compote.

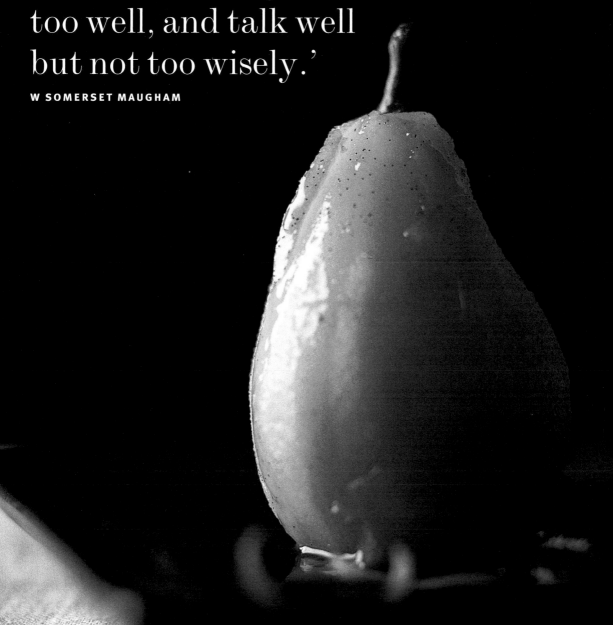

'At a dinner party one should eat wisely but not too well, and talk well but not too wisely.'

W SOMERSET MAUGHAM

Menu Two

Tom yam kung

This flavoursome Thai prawn and mushroom soup is sure to impress your dinner party guests. You can adjust the amount of chilli according to your taste. Shiitake mushrooms have powerful immunity and healing properties and are also believed to help ease numerous conditions, from colds and flu to gastrointestinal problems.

SERVES 4
30ml (2 tbsp) groundnut or sunflower oil
2 shallots (or 1 small onion), peeled and chopped
5cm (2in) piece fresh root ginger, chopped
2 garlic cloves, peeled and chopped
30ml (2 tbsp) chilli sauce
1 litre (1³/₄ pints) vegetable stock
1 lemongrass stalk, lightly crushed
5ml (1 tsp) demerara sugar
16 tiger prawns, shelled, deveined
125g (4oz) shiitake mushrooms
Juice of 1 lime
Small handful fresh coriander leaves, roughly chopped

1 Heat the oil in a large pan, add the shallots, ginger and garlic and sauté over a gentle heat for 2 or 3 minutes.
2 Add the chilli sauce, stock, lemongrass and sugar. Bring to the boil, then reduce the heat and simmer for 10 minutes.
3 Add the mushrooms and prawns and cook for a few minutes.
4 Add the lime juice, then ladle into bowls. Scatter the coriander leaves over and serve.

Pan-fried tuna on cannellini beans with rice noodles

Fresh tuna (not the tinned version) is rich in Omega-3 oils, which help keep the skin smooth and supple, as well as prevent heart attacks and stroke, and alleviate inflammatory conditions such as arthritis. Cannellini beans, while full of fibre, magnesium and iron, can look quite dull on their own, so it's important to combine them with colourful ingredients, such as cherry tomatoes and rocket, as in this recipe.

SERVES 4
30ml (2 tbsp) olive oil
2 garlic cloves, crushed
400g (14 oz) tinned cannellini beans, drained
125g (4 oz) cherry tomatoes
Juice and zest of 1 lemon
4 x 150g (5 oz) tuna steaks
225g (8 oz) rice vermicelli noodles
A drizzle of sesame oil
A handful of rocket

1 Heat the olive oil in a non-stick frying pan, add the garlic and cook for 1 minute. Add the beans, tomatoes and lemon juice and zest. Warm over a low heat for 5 minutes.
2 Brush the tuna steaks with a little olive oil. Heat a non-stick pan until hot. Add the tuna and fry for 2–3 minutes, turn over and cook the other side for 3 minutes. Remove from the heat.
3 Put the noodles in a bowl, cover with boiling water and let them soak for 5 minutes. Drain and rinse under cold running water. Transfer to a bowl, sprinkle with the sesame oil and stir briefly to coat.
4 Pile the noodles onto four serving plates, place the beans on top and scatter over the rocket. Top with the tuna steaks and serve immediately.

Warm figs with raspberry sorbet

Fresh figs are real nutritional powerhouses – they contain mood-relaxing serotonin as well as fibre, potassium and beta-carotene. Here they are poached with port and red wine, both good sources of heart-protective flavonoids but you can substitute red grape juice (without losing the heart-friendly nutrients) if you prefer. The raspberry sorbet is an excellent way of boosting your vitamin-C intake, and this version contains only half the sugar of traditional recipes.

SERVES 4
100g (3^1/$_2$ oz) caster sugar
150ml (5fl oz) water
150ml (5fl oz) apple juice
700g (1^1/$_2$ lb) raspberries (fresh or frozen)
60ml (2fl oz) lime or lemon juice
2.5cm (1in) cinnamon stick
1 glass (150ml/5fl oz) port
2 glasses (300ml/5fl oz) red wine
85g (3oz) dark brown sugar
8 fresh figs

1 Put the sugar, water and juice in a heavy-based saucepan over a low heat and stir until the sugar has dissolved. Increase the heat and boil for 5 minutes. Set aside to cool.

2 Place the raspberries and lime or lemon juice in a food processor and whiz to a smooth purée. Press through a fine sieve to remove the seeds, rubbing the mixture through with the back of a wooden spoon. Combine the fruit purée and syrup. Churn in an ice cream maker until almost frozen solid, then transfer into a plastic container and put in the freezer until you are ready to serve.

3 Put the cinnamon stick, port, wine and brown sugar in a pan. Bring to the boil and cook until reduced and thickened into a syrup. Add the figs and poach for 5 minutes, until tender. Remove with a slotted spoon and serve the figs warm with a scoop of sorbet.

Skin food

Food is good for our insides; it can do wonders for our outsides too. Food doesn't just have to be for eating – why not take a leaf out of Poppea's book and feed your skin from the outside at the same time?

If you or a friend are a dab hand at massage, then so much the better. Massage is a great way to unwind, relax and get rid of that harmful (and ageing) stress hormone, cortisol. A gentle massage on your face helps tone the skin, and clear toxins and waste; it boosts circulation to bring a rejuvenating glow to your skin and it can make you look more alive, healthy and young.

'Milk is valued for giving a part of its whiteness to the skin of women. Poppea, wife of Domitius Nero, took 500 nursing asses everywhere in her travelling party, and soaked herself completely in a bath of this milk, in the belief that it would make her skin more supple.'

PLINY, WRITING IN THE FIRST CENTURY AD

Food for the face

Before you put on a face mask, cover your skin with a thin layer of gauze. Apply the mask over it. You will still get the benefit of the ingredients but, when you've finished, it's much quicker (and cleaner) to get the mask off.

⋯⟩ The skin round our eyes is extremely delicate and can be one of the first places to show signs of ageing. To keep the years at bay, you want firm, wrinkle-free skin. Cucumber is great for cooling and de-puffing the skin round the eyes. Grate some cucumber and pop it in the fridge. Then wrap the cucumber in some gauze and pop over your eyes or irritated skin and lie back and relax. (Grated potato can also be used in the same way.)

⋯⟩ Chamomile tea bags can also cool tired, puffy eyes.

⋯⟩ Cucumber and yogurt, blended together, are an effective face mask that can perk up tired, old-looking skin.

⋯⟩ As we get older, cell renewal slows down so skin can look dull, tired and, frankly, old. Oats and honey mixed together are a great facial exfoliator (honey is a healer and an antiseptic; oats balance the oils of the skin) to bring out a gorgeous glow.

⋯⟩ Or mix 2 tablespoons of oats and 1 tablespoon of sweet almond oil together for a gentle face scrub.

⋯⟩ Don't forget to exfoliate your elbows; that wrinkly dry skin is a dead giveaway for looking ancient.

⋯⟩ Light vegetable oils (grapeseed or avocado oil) are good for body, hair, nail and cuticle conditioning.

⋯⟩ Massage skin with some avocado oil which is a wonderful source of vitamin E (ideal for ironing out wrinkles). Or mash up an avocado, mix with live yogurt and spread on your face. Massage over face, working the pressure points between the brows, at the temples, along the jawline and on the earlobes. Great work-out for your facial muscles and a marvellous stress-buster.

⋯⟩ Rub the inside of the avocado skin over your elbows and knees to get rid of that wrinkly-elephant look.

⋯⟩ For a fruity moisturizer, blend a little banana with some milk. Massage over your face and leave for 20 minutes.

Food for the hands

After your face and neck, the hands are the next to suffer the tell-tale signs of ageing. Exfoliate your hands with a mixture of olive oil and granulated sugar.

⋯> The skin on our hands takes a battering from day to day: hot water, bright sun, cold wind can all strip the moisture from our skin and leave us with old, dry wrinkly hands. Keep the skin supple and moisturized by making your own hand cream. Take some hemp oil (which is rich in Omega-3 and -6 essential oils) or olive oil (a traditional Mediterranean moisturizer, rich in Omega-9) and mix with petroleum jelly. Rub the mixture into your hands and then cover them with freezer bags. Sit back and enjoy some music or a bit of gossip with a friend while your hands get the full moisturizing benefit.

⋯> Alternatively, almond oil is great for softening and soothing the skin, helping to prevent stretch marks and scarring. Massage a few drops onto the back of your hands and into your nails. It also improves your cuticles and helps nail growth.

⋯> Hands that are stained or discoloured don't project an image of youth and loveliness. To get rid of the marks, rub half a cut lemon over them. Rinse your hands carefully, then apply a moisturizer because the lemon can have a drying effect on the skin.

⋯> Rubbing a potato over your hands also gets rid of marks. Make sure you rinse your hands afterwards before applying a moisturizer.

⋯> If you start to get white spots on your nails, your diet may be low in zinc so you need to up your levels (see page 35 for zinc-rich foods).

'Don't put anything on your face that you wouldn't put in your mouth.' HELENA RUBINSTEIN

Food for the feet

We've been concentrating on the face a lot but don't forget your feet. If they feel good, so do you. For a great foot-bath, quarter fill a washing-up bowl with warm water and add a few drops of essential oil, diluted in a cup of alcohol. Lavender is soothing, while rosemary, peppermint and thyme are all pick-me-ups.

For a foot mask, use a face mask. Yes, whatever you put on your face will work just as well on your feet. Why should they be left out?

'I'm tired of all this nonsense about beauty being only skin deep. That's deep enough. What do you want, an adorable pancreas?' JEAN KERR

Store cupboard stand-bys

Thinking ahead and planning your meals is a great way to make sure you are including as many super foods in your diet as possible. A rumbling tummy and an empty fridge or cupboard can be dangerous – you find yourself reaching for the phone to dial for a pizza or rushing off to the supermarket to grab an instant meal. With a well-stocked larder and fridge, you should never find yourself caught short and able to whip up a delicious, anti-ageing meal at any time.

Fridge
- Milk, skimmed
- Low-fat live yogurt
- Avocados
- Peppers (red, green, yellow, orange)
- Carrots
- Green veg, such as broccoli, spinach, cauliflower, cabbage
- Tomatoes
- Beetroot
- Lettuce
- Fresh fruit, such as mangoes, guava, melon, blueberries, raspberries, blackberries, cranberries
- Skinless chicken and turkey breast
- Fish (ideally eat it fresh; otherwise store in the freezer)

Larder
- Canned fish (in water, not oil: salmon, sardines, tuna, mackerel, anchovies)
- Free-range eggs
- Porridge oats
- Oatcakes
- Brown rice
- Dried/canned pulses and lentils (chickpeas, kidney beans, baked beans, barley, millet)
- Honey, ideally Manuka
- Oils (extra-virgin olive oil, rapeseed/ flaxseed oil)
- Olives
- Onions
- Garlic
- Ginger
- Sweet potatoes
- Fresh fruits, such as apples, oranges, lots of lemons, bananas, grapes, berries, kiwi fruit – whatever is in season
- Tinned fruit, such as guava, papaya
- Dried apricots, raisins, figs, prunes
- Nuts (almonds, walnuts, brazil nuts) and seeds (including sesame, pumpkin and flax seeds)
- Peanut butter
- Canned tomatoes
- Tea – herbal, green, rooibos
- Pomegranate juice

On the kitchen windowsill
- Basil
- Parsley

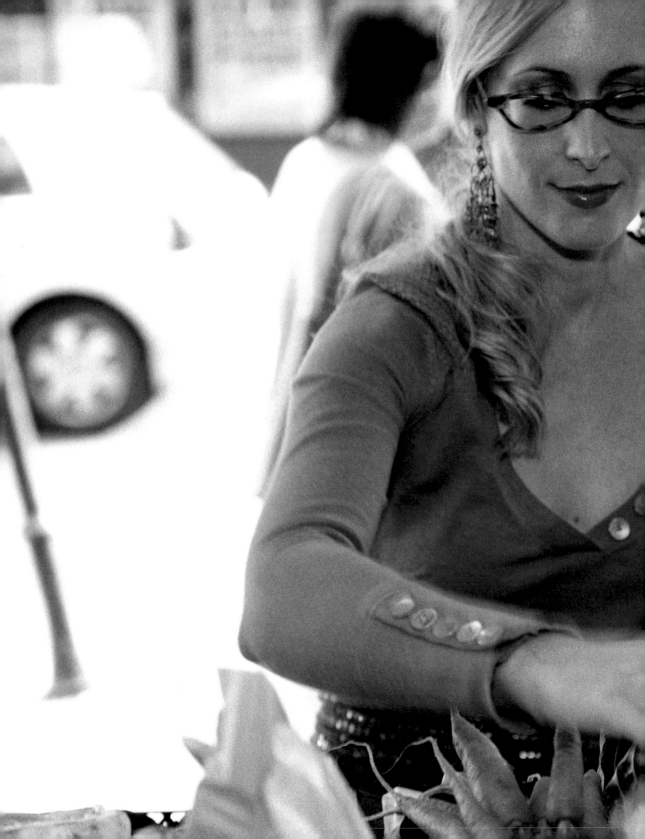

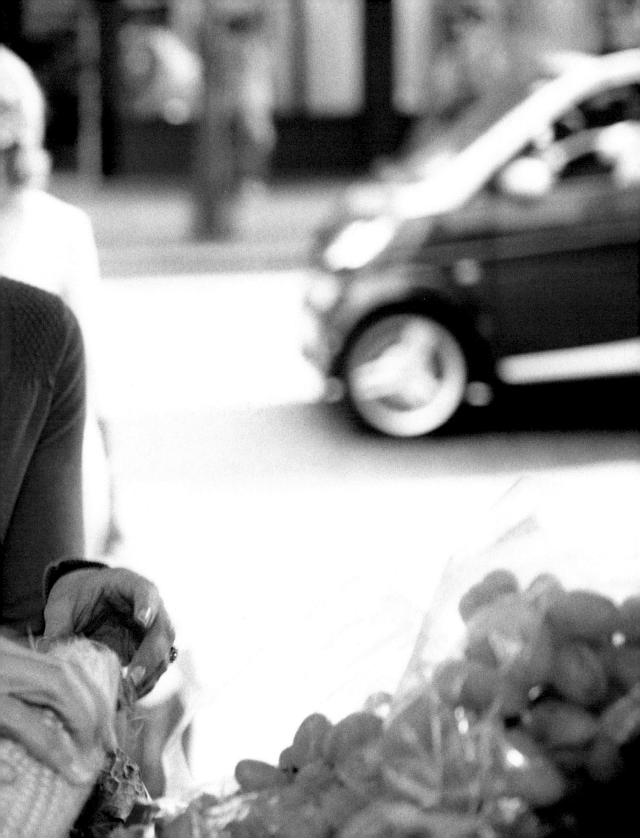

Food sources for vitamins, minerals and other nutrients

Vitamins

Vitamin A (also known as retinol)
Found in animal food sources including:
Butter
Cheese (though not low-fat varieties)
Egg yolks
Fish liver oils (particularly cod and halibut fish oils)
Kidneys
Liver
Meat
Milk
Oily fish (such as salmon, mackerel, herring, trout)

Beta carotene (converted by the body into vitamin A)
Food sources are orange, yellow and green fruits and vegetables including:
Apricots and peaches
Asparagus
Cantaloupe melon
Carrots
Dark green leafy vegetables (such as broccoli, cabbage, Brussels sprouts, spinach, watercress)
Green beans
Leeks
Mangoes
Parsley
Peas
Red and yellow peppers
Papayas
Pink grapefruit
Plums
Pumpkins and squash
Sweet potatoes

Vitamin B complex
B1 (thiamin)
Brewer's yeast
Brown rice
Egg yolks
Fish (especially salmon)
Legumes
Liver
Nuts
Poultry
Pulses
Seaweed (kelp)
Spirulina
Wheatgerm
Whole grains

B2 (riboflavin)
Cheese
Eggs
Fish
Green leafy vegetables (such as broccoli, cabbage, spinach, watercress)
Lean meat
Legumes
Milk
Nuts (including almonds and walnuts)
Wholegrains
Yogurt

B3 (niacin)
Beetroot
Brewer's yeast
Fish (including salmon, tuna, cod, halibut)
Liver
Meat (including chicken, turkey, pork)
Liver
Nuts (particularly almonds, hazelnuts, peanuts)
Sunflower seeds
Yogurt

B5 (pantothenic acid)
Almonds
Avocados
Beef
Brewer's yeast
Cauliflower
Cereals
Chicken
Corn
Egg yolks
Fish and shellfish (including lobster and salmon)
Green leafy vegetables (especially broccoli and kale)
Legumes
Lentils (and other pulses such as chick peas)
Meat (particularly beef and liver)
Milk
Poultry (including chicken, duck, turkey)
Soy beans
Sweet potatoes
Wheatgerm
Wholegrains

B6 (pyridoxine)
Avocados
Bananas
Brewer's yeast
Brown rice
Carrots
Chicken and turkey
Eggs
Fish (especially salmon, shrimp, tuna)
Lentils
Liver
Nuts (particularly walnuts)
Peas
Soy beans
Sunflower seeds
Walnuts
Wheatgerm
Whole grain flour

B12 (cobalamin)
Dairy products
Eggs
Fish (especially halibut and salmon)
Meat (in particular beef, kidney, liver, pork)
Yogurt

Folate (folic acid)
Asparagus
Avocados
Beetroot
Cauliflower
Dried beans
Green leafy vegetables (such as Brussels sprouts, cabbage, kale, spring greens, spinach)
Legumes
Oranges (and other citrus fruits)
Parsnips
Wheatgerm

Vitamin C
The main sources are fresh fruit and vegetables. The richest include:
Fruit:
Blackcurrants
Citrus fruit (especially grapefruits, oranges and tangerines)
Guava
Kiwi fruit
Lychees
Mangoes

Melons (cantaloupe, honeydew, watermelon)
Nectarines
Papaya
Pawpaw
Persimmons
Raspberries
Rosehips
Strawberries
Tomatoes
Vegetables:
Broccoli
Brussels sprouts
Cabbage
Cauliflower
Cucumbers
Kale
Mangetout
Peas
Peppers
Potatoes
Spinach
Spring greens
Watercress

Vitamin D
Dairy products (including butter, cheese, margarine, milk)
Eggs
Fish liver oils (especially cod and halibut)
Liver
Oily fish (including mackerel, sardines, salmon, tuna)
Sunlight
Yogurt

Vitamin E
Avocados
Blackberries
Mangoes
Nuts (particularly almonds, hazelnuts, pecans)
Olives
Seeds (especially sunflower)
Spinach
Sweet potatoes
Tomatoes
Vegetable oils (including corn, olive, sunflower)
Watercress
Wheatgerm
Whole grain cereals

Minerals

Calcium
Canned bony fish (such as mackerel, pilchards, sardines, salmon, tuna)
Dairy products (including milk and cheese)
Dried apricots and figs
Green leafy vegetables (such as broccoli, kale, spinach, watercress)
Nuts (especially almonds, brazil nuts, hazelnuts)
Okra
Oysters
Pulses
Seaweed
Sesame seeds
Tofu
Wheatgerm
Yogurt

Chromium
Brewer's yeast
Beef
Calves' liver
Chicken
Eggs
Nuts
Oysters
Peppers
Whole grains

Iron
Dark chocolate
Dried fruit (especially apricots, figs, raisins, prunes)
Egg yolks
Green leafy vegetables (including broccoli, cabbage, kale, spinach, watercress)
Lean red meat (including game)
Legumes (beans and peas)
Lentils
Liver and kidneys
Nuts (particularly almonds)
Oily fish (such as mackerel, sardines, tuna)
Oysters
Whole grains

Magnesium
Avocados
Bananas
Brown rice
Dried fruit (especially apricots and figs)

Green leafy vegetables
Legumes
Nuts
Oats
Okra
Parsnips
Pulses
Seeds
Soy beans
Tofu
Whole grains (including cereals and bread)
Yogurt

Potassium
Bananas (and some other fruit including apricots, kiwi, melon)
Dried fruit (especially apricots and prunes)
Fish
Oranges (particularly the juice)
Potatoes
Poultry
Spinach
Squash
Tomatoes

Selenium
Brazil nuts
Cashew nuts
Cereals
Cheese
Chicken
Eggs
Fish (including shellfish)
Lean meat
Milk
Seaweed
Sunflower seeds
Walnuts
Whole wheat

Silica
Barley
Beetroot
Horsetail herb
Millet
Oats
Onions
Whole wheat

Sulphur
Broccoli
Brussels sprouts
Cabbage
Horseradish root

Zinc
Cheese (particularly hard cheeses like Parmesan)
Egg yolks
Fish
Lean meat (including beef, lamb, venison)
Liver and kidneys
Milk
Mushrooms
Nuts
Poultry (chicken, duck, goose, turkey)
Pulses
Sardines
Seeds
Shellfish (especially crab, oysters, lobster, mussels)
Wheatgerm
Wholegrains

Essential fatty acids

Omega-3
Avocados
Cold water oily fish (especially anchovies, herring, mackerel, sardines, salmon, tuna)
Canned fish (sardines, salmon, tuna)
Dark green leafy vegetables (for instance, broccoli, kale and spinach contain the alpha-linolenic acid [ALA] type of omega-3)
Flax (also known as linseeds), hemp and pumpkin seeds, and their oils
Scallops
Seaweed
Pecans
Walnuts (and walnut oil)

Omega-6
Canned fish (sardines and tuna)
Cereals
Eggs
Flax, hemp and pumpkin seeds, and their oils
Nuts (especially almonds, brazil nuts, hazelnuts, peanuts, pecans, pine nuts, pistachios, walnuts)
Poultry
Sesame seeds
Vegetable oils (including corn, rapeseed [or canola], safflower, soya, sunflower. Although good sources, these are often refined

and so nutrient deficient as sold in many stores)

Gamma Linolenic Acid (GLA)
(This is an Omega-6 essential fatty acid)
Blackcurrant seed oil
Borage oil
Evening primrose oil

Omega-9
(Not strictly an essential fatty acid)
Avocados
Nuts (including almonds, hazelnuts, peanuts)
Olive oil
Olives
Sesame seeds and their oil

Proteins

Essential amino acids
(Animal sources contain all the essential amino acids)
Dairy products
Eggs
Fish and shellfish
Lean meat (including game and venison)
Poultry (especially chicken and turkey)
(Plant-based sources don't contain all the essential amino acids unless taken in combination – the exception is soya)
Legumes
Lentils (and other pulses)
Nuts
Seeds (including pumpkin, sesame, sunflower)
Soya
Wheatgerm
Whole grains (including oats, rice, quinoa)

Nucleic acids
Asparagus
Bran
Chicken liver
Fish (especially anchovies, salmon, sardines)
Mushrooms
Oatmeal
Onions
Spinach
Wheatgerm

Directory

Allergies & Conditions

Action Against Allergy
PO Box 278
Twickenham TW1 4QQ
Tel: 0208 892 2711
www.actionagainstallergy.freeserve.co.uk

Allergy UK
3 White Oak Square
London Road
Swanley
Kent BR8 7AG
Tel: 01322 619898 / allergy helpline:
01322 619864
www.allergyfoundation.com

Anaphylaxis Campaign
PO Box 275
Farnborough
Hampshire GU14 6SX
Tel: 01252 542029
www.anaphylaxis.org.uk

British Heart Foundation
14 Fitzhardinge Street
London W1H 6DH
Tel: 020 7935 0185
www.bhf.org.uk

The Coeliac Society
PO Box 220
High Wycombe
Buckinghamshire HP11 2HY
Tel: 01494 437278
www.coeliac.co.uk

Diabetes UK
Central Office
10 Parkway
London NW1 7AA
Tel: 020 7424 1000
www.diabetes.org.uk

Digestive Disorders Foundation
3 St Andrews Place
London NW1 4LB
Tel: 020 7486 0341
www.digestivedisorders.org.uk

National Eczema Society
Hill House
Highgate Hill
London N19 5NA
Tel: 020 7281 3553; helpline
0870 241 3604 (Mon–Fri 8am–8pm)
www.eczema.org

National Osteoporisis Society
PO Box 10
Radstock
Bath BA3 3YB
Tel: 01761 471771 (general enquiries)
Helpline: 01761 472721 (medical queries)
www.nos.org.uk

The YorkTest Food Scan Intolerance Test
Tel: 0800 074 6145
www.yorktest.com

Diet

Vegan Society UK
Donald Watson House
7 Battle Road
St Leonards-on-Sea
East Sussex TN37 7AA
Tel: 01424 427 393
www.vegansociety.com

Vegetarian Society of the UK
Parkdale
Dunham Road
Altrincham
Cheshire WA14 4QG
Tel: 0161 928 0793
www.vegsoc.org

Food – general

British Cheese Board
Dragon Court
27 Macklin Street
London WC2B 5LX
Tel: 0117 921 1744
www.britishcheese.com

British Egg Information Service
Bury House
126–128 Cromwell Road
London SW7 4ET
www.britegg.co.uk

British Potato Council
4300 Nash Court
John Smith Drive
Oxford Business Park
Oxford OX4 2RT
Tel: 01865 714455
www.potato.org.uk

Canned Food Information Service
Vincent House
Tindle Bridge
92–93 Edward Street
Birmingham B1 2RA
Tel: 0800 243 364
www.cannedfood.co.uk

CIWF (Compassion in World Farming)
Charles House
5a Charles Street
Petersfield
Hampshire GU32 3EH
Tel: 01730 264 208
www.ciwf.org.uk

The Dairy Council
5–7 John Princes Street
London W1M 0AP
Tel: 020 7499 7822
www.milk.co.uk

DEFRA (Department of Environment, Farming & Rural Affairs)
Information Resource Centre
Lower Ground Floor
Ergon House
c/o Nobel House
17 Smith Square
London SW1P 3JR
Tel: 08459 33 55 77 (helpline)
www.defra.gov.uk

Federation of Bakers
6 Catherine Street
London WC2B 5JW
Tel: 020 7420 7190
www.bakersfederation.org.uk

Flour Advisory Bureau
21 Arlington Street
London SW1A 1RN
Tel: 020 7493 2521
www.fabflour.co.uk

Food and Drink Federation
6 Catherine Street
London WC2B 5JJ
Tel: 020 7836 2460
www.foodfitness.org.uk

The Food Commission
94 White Lion Street
London N1 9PF
Tel: 020 7837 2250
www.foodcomm.org.uk
(Independent food watchdog campaigning
for safer, healthier food in the UK)

Food Safety Authority of Ireland
Abbey Court
Lower Abbey Street
Dublin 1
Ireland
Tel: +353 1 817 1300
www.fsai.ie
(Consumer advice on food storage,
shopping and cooking processes)

Food Standards Agency
Room 6/21 Hannibal House
PO Box 30080
Elephant & Castle
London SE1 6YA
Tel: 0845 757 3012
www.food.gov.uk
(Independent and balanced advice on food
safety)

Friends of the Earth
26–28 Underwood Street
London N1 7JQ
Tel: 0808 800 1111 (information service)
www.foe.co.uk

Frozen Food Information Service
c/o Fox Publishing
1st Floor, Lion House
1 Red Lion Street
Richmond
Surrey TW9 1RE
Tel: 020 8940 4063
www.bfff.co.uk/factfall.htm

Marine Conservation Society
Unit 3
Wolf Business Park
Alton Road
Ross-on-Wye
Herefordshire HR9 5NB
Tel: 01989 566017
www.mcsuk.org
www.fishonline.org
(For everything you need to know about
fishing policy and which fish to eat)

Scottish Food & Drink
Tel: 0845 601 3752
www.scottishfoodanddrink.com
Email: info@scottishfoodanddrink.com

Seafish (The Sea Fish Industry Authority)
18 Logie Mill
Logie Green Road
Edinburgh EH7 4HS
Tel: 0131 558 3331
www.seafish.org
(Promotes good-quality, sustainable
seafood; lots of fish recipes)

The Sugar Bureau
Duncan House
Dolphin Square
London SW1V 3PW
Tel: 020 7823 9465
www.sugar-bureau.co.uk
(To improve knowledge and understanding
about the contributions of sugar and other
carbohydrates)

General Health

Department of Health
Richmond House
79 Whitehall
London SW1A 2NL
Tel: 020 7210 4850
www.doh.gov.uk

Food Education Board for Scotland
Woodburn House
Canaan Lane
Edinburgh EH10 4SG
Tel: 0131 536 5500
www.hebs.scot.nhs.uk/topics/diet/
index.htm

Nutrition

British Association for Nutritional Therapy
27 Gloucester Street
London WC1N 3XX
Tel: 0870 6061284
(Send £2 + large SAE for a list of registered
nutritional therapists)

British Nutrition Foundation
High Holborn House
52–54 High Holborn
London WC1 6RQ
Tel: 020 7404 6504
www.nutrition.org.uk

Institute for Optimum Nutrition
Blades Court
Deodar Road
London SW15 2NU
Tel: 020 8877 9993
www.ion.ac.uk

The Nutrition Society
10 Cambridge Court
210 Shepherd's Bush Road
London W6 7NJ
Tel: 020 7602 0228
www.nutsoc.org.uk

The Natural Health Advisory Service
PO Box 268
Lewes
Sussex BN7 2QN
Tel: 01273 487366
www.naturalhealthas.com
(now incorporates the Women's Nutritional
Advisory Service)

Organic

**Irish Organic Farmers & Growers
Association**
Main Street
Newtownforbes
Co. Longford
Eire
Tel: (+353) 043 42495
www.irishorganic.ie

Organic Consumers Association
6771 South Silver Hill Drive
Finland MN 55603
USA
www.organicconsumers.org

The UK Organic Directory
www.organicliving.ukf.net

The Soil Association
Bristol House
40–56 Victoria Street
Bristol BS1 6BY
Tel: 0117 929 0661
www.soilassociation.org

Shopping for Food

FARMA (the National Farmers' Retail and Markets Association)
PO Box 575
Southampton SO15 7BZ
Tel: 0845 45 88 420
www.farmersmarkets.net

Farm Shops
The Farm Retail Association
Tel: 0845 230 2150
www.farmshopping.com
(Now part of FARMA)

London Farmers' Markets
11 O'Donnell Court
Brunswick Centre
London WC1N 1NY
Tel: 020 7833 0338
www.lfm.org.uk

The Scottish Association of Farmers' Markets
www.scottishfarmersmarkets.co.uk

Supplements

Consumers for Health Choice
Southbank House
Black Prince Road
London SE1 7SJ
Tel: 020 7463 0690
www.healthchoice.org.uk
(Provides up-to-date information on regulations concerning supplements and herbals remedies)

GNC Live Well
www.gnc.co.uk
(Online shopping)

Victoria Health
Tel: 0800 389 8195
www.victoriahealth.com
(Online shopping and information on health matters)

Vegetable & Fruit Box Schemes

Able and Cole
Tel: 0845 262 6262
www.abel-cole.co.uk

Fair Organics
Tel: 01277 890188
www.fairorganics.co.uk

Farmaround
Tel: 020 7627 8066
www.farmaround.co.uk

Riverford Organic Vegetables
Tel: 0845 600 2311
www.riverford.co.uk

Sunnyfields Organic
Tel: 02380 861266
www.sunnyfields.co.uk

Women's Health

British Menopause Society
4–6 Eton Place
Marlow
Buckinghamshire SL7 2QA
Tel: 01628 890199
www.the-bms.org
(For professionals working in the field)

The Daisy Network
PO Box 183
Rossendale BB4 6WZ
www.daisynetwork.org.uk
(For women suffering from premature menopause – before the age of 40)

Early Menopause
www.earlymenopause.com
(American website)

The Menopause Amarant Trust
80 Lambeth Road
London SE1 7PW
Tel: 01293 413000 (Mon–Fri 11am–6pm)
www.amarantmenopausetrust.org.uk
(Charity set up to promote a better understanding of the menopause and greater awareness of the benefits of HRT)

Museum of Menstruation & Women's Health
www.mum.org

The National Association for Premenstrual Syndrome (NAPS)
41 Old Road
East Peckham
Kent TN12 5AP
Tel: 0870 777 2178
E: contact@pms.org.uk
www.pms.org.uk

The Natural Menopause Advice Service
PO Box 71
Leatherhead
Surrey KT22 7DP
www.nmas.org.uk

Women's Health
52 Featherstone Street
London EC1 8RT
Tel: 020 7251 6333; helpline 0845 125 5254
(Mon–Fri 9.30am–1.30pm)

Women's Health Concern
10 Storey's Gate
London SW1P 3AY
Tel: 020 7799 9897
www.womens-health-concern.org

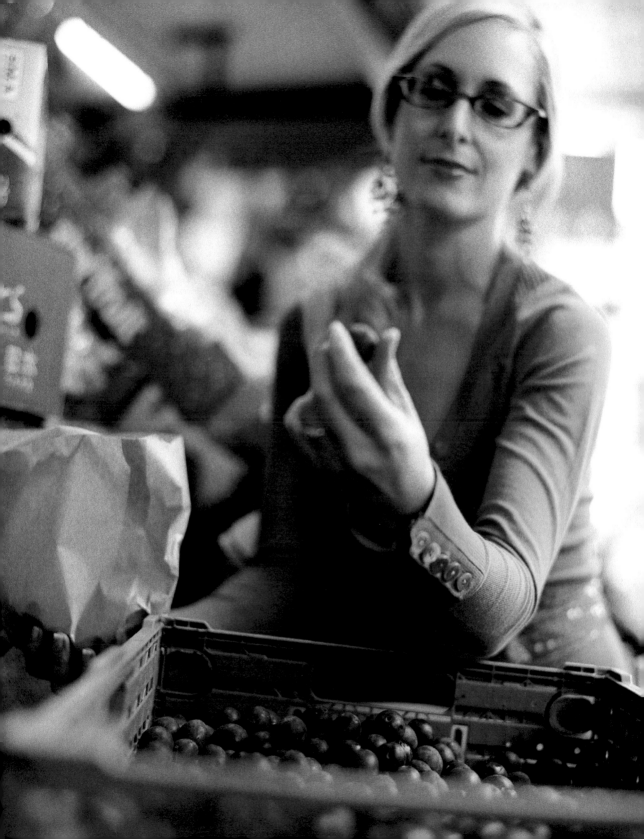

Index

(Individual recipes are listed under main recipes entry)

About the author

Nicky Hambleton-Jones is a qualified dietician and ran a nutrition practice in her native South Africa before moving to London in 1996. After spending four years working as a management consultant in the City, she decided she was far more passionate about fashion and in 2001 she established Tramp2Vamp.

Tramp2Vamp (www.tramp2vamp.com) is a style consultancy which helps people to look fantastic effortlessly, whether you're stuck in a rut and need a complete overhaul or you're simply looking for that fabulous outfit for a special occasion. 'Each and every one of us has the potential to look good, every day of our lives; my clients certainly do.'

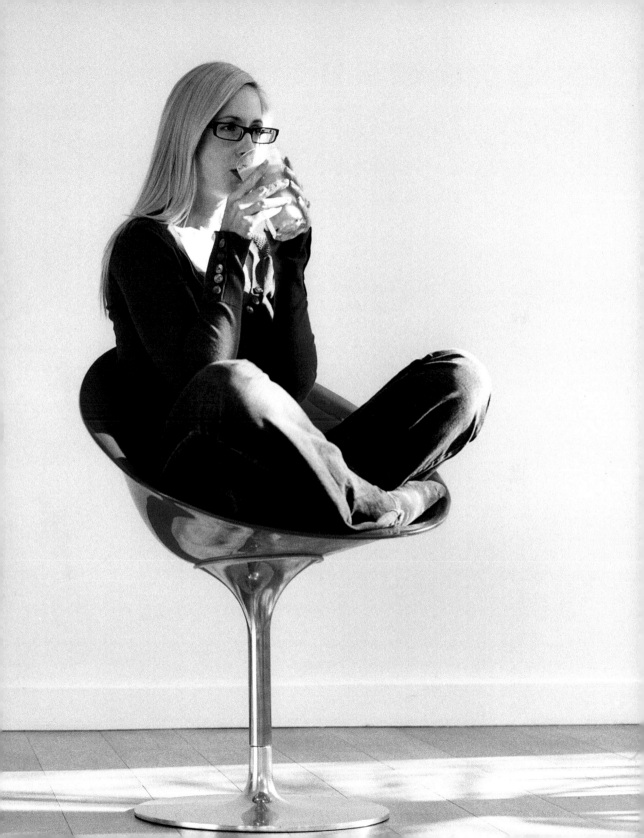

Author's acknowledgements

I would like to thank Karen Dolby and Katherine Lapworth for all their hard work and perseverance in pulling the material for this book together. It wasn't easy, but the end result is fantastic.

I'd also like to thank Alex, Emma and Saskia from Smith & Gilmour for making work so much fun and for producing such beautiful results. And my favourite photographer Mark Read for eternally making me look 10 years younger! Where would I be without you?

Thanks to everyone at Maverick and especially Colette Foster for her enthusiasm and support. To Helen Pope, our tireless researcher, for her humour, efficiency and resourcefulness. Last, but not least, the team at Transworld and in particular, Doug Young, Sarah Emsley and Gillian Haslam – thank you for everything.

Quite simply, the book wouldn't have happened without you all.

The publishers would like to thank Collins of Chiswick, Chiswick High Rd, London and Fish Works, Turnham Green Terrace, London, www.fishworks.co.uk for allowing us to take photographs at their fantastic locations.